Acute and Transient Psychoses

T0172119

Brief and acute psychotic disorders with a short duration and a generally good prognosis have long intrigued psychiatrists. Although they are included in internationally accepted diagnostic systems, understanding of these disorders remains minimal. This book is the first comprehensive overview of the clinical features, biology, course and long-term outcome of brief and acute psychoses. The authors review the world literature on the topic and they also present data from their own longitudinal study – the most complete investigation of this group of disorders so far conducted. The book concludes with considerations of the nosological status of brief and acute psychoses and their impact on our understanding of the continuum of psychotic and affective disorders.

The authors are based at the Martin-Luther-Universität of Halle-Wittenberg, Germany.

Andreas Marneros is Professor of Psychiatry in the Department of Psychiatry and Psychotherapy and **Frank Pillmann** is Specialist Psychiatrist there. Professor Marneros won the Kraepelin Research Prize in 2002 for his work in the psychoses, especially schizoaffective and acute brief psychoses.

Acute and Transient Psychoses

Andreas Marneros and Frank Pillmann

Martin-Luther-Universität, Halle-Wittenberg, Germany

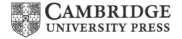

CAMBRIDGE
UNIVERSITY PRESS

CAMBRIDGE UNIVERSITY PRESS
Cambridge, New York, Melbourne, Madrid, Cape Town, Singapore, São Paulo, Delhi

Cambridge University Press
The Edinburgh Building, Cambridge CB2 8RU, UK

Published in the United States of America by Cambridge University Press, New York

www.cambridge.org
Information on this title: www.cambridge.org/9780521114066

First published 2004
This digitally printed version 2009

A catalogue record for this publication is available from the British Library

Library of Congress Cataloguing in Publication data
Marneros, A. (Andreas), 1946 – Acute and Transient Psychoses/by Andreas Marneros and Frank Pillmann.
    p.   cm.
    Includes bibliographical references and index.
    ISBN 0 521 83518 6 (hardback: alk. paper)
    1. Psychoses. I. Title: Acute and transient psychoses. II. Pillmann, Frank, 1961 – III. Title.
    [DNLM: 1. Psychotic Disorders. 2. Acute Disease. 3. Longitudinal Studies. WM 200 M353b 2003]
    RC512.M376 2003
    616.89 – dc22   2003062530

ISBN 978-0-521-83518-3 hardback
ISBN 978-0-521-11406-6 paperback

No one with experience will deny that the cases are upsettingly frequent in which, despite the most careful clinical observation, it seems impossible to arrive at a definite judgement [with regard to the differentiation of manic-depressive illness and dementia praecox].

Emil Kraepelin 1920

The nomenclature of these acute disorders is as uncertain as their nosological status [. . .]. Systematic clinical information that would provide definitive guidance on the classification of acute psychotic disorders is not yet available, and the limited data and clinical tradition that must therefore be used instead do not give rise to concepts that can be clearly defined and separated from each other.

World Health Organization 1992

Contents

Preface

The road to the modern definitions of Brief and Acute Psychoses has been very long. Efforts to define and understand such brief, acute and good prognosis psychoses are very old-fashioned. Certainly, the definitions of ICD-10 for 'Acute and Transient Psychotic Disorders' and that of DSM-IV for 'Brief Psychotic Disorder' are not unchangeable and are also not final diagnoses. It could be assumed that even the present diagnostic algorithms will be changed. The main reason for the expected changes is that only very little and unsystematic research on this topic exists. We know really very little about the clinical aspects, the precipitants or the longitudinal prognosis. We hardly know anything about their aetiology, biology and genetics. But the relevance of such brief, acute, transient, good prognosis or 'atypical' psychoses for researchers and for clinicians is clear. No serious biological, genetic, pharmacological, prognostic and clinical research is possible if we do not have exact definitions or if we do not have exactly defined homogeneous groups of patients. Voluminous, diffuse and elastic groups of mental disorders called schizophrenia or affective disorders are a main handicap for effective research. But we also need exact clinical diagnoses and psychopathological understanding of the so-called 'atypical psychoses' because of clinical, therapeutic and prognostic aspects affecting long-term plans of patients and their relatives. Future research must seek aetiological, biological or genetic similarities and differences between the 'atypical' and 'typical' psychoses. This book might be a contribution to such efforts.

Acknowledgements

This book would not have been possible without the valuable help of a number of colleagues at Halle-Wittenberg University Hospital who were involved in various stages of the Halle Study on Brief and Acute Psychoses (HASBAP). The authors thank Dr Annette Haring, Dr Sabine Balzuweit, Dipl.-Psych. Raffaela Blöink, Dr Andrea Wenzel, Dr Stefan Röttig, Dr Thomas Arndt, Dr Ursel Sannemüller Dr Rolf Spindler, Dr Michaela Nagel, Cand. Med. Juliane Wünsche and Cand. Med. Daniel Radler for their assistance in many tasks of data acquisition and data analysis. Our thanks extend to Ina Nelles for the skilful preparation of the manuscript and to Frank Demel for his help with the pictures.

The HASBAP was supported by a grant of the German Research Council (DFG MA 115/12-1). The authors also gratefully acknowledge this support.

We also thank the patients who willingly, openly and repeatedly participated in the follow-up investigations.

Part I

History and concepts

Psychiatric sculptors and psychiatric sculptures: the unformed clay and Kraepelin's visions

The efforts to define homogenous groups of mental disorders are very similar to the work of a sculptor. The artist usually has to cut small, but also sometimes larger, pieces of wood, marble or clay in an attempt to give the material an identifiable feature. But the material that has been cut continues to exist, not as part of the sculpture, but as material left in the sculptor's workshop.

The history of psychiatry from ancient times to the present is full of the efforts of scientists to create identifiable diagnostic groups (Leibrand and Wettley, 1961; Alexander and Selesnick, 1966; Ackerknecht, 1968; Marneros and Angst, 2000; Angst and Marneros, 2001). But the material of the psychiatric sculptor is not similar to marble or wood, but rather similar to clay. Psychiatrists usually change the form of the diagnosis like the artist the shape of the clay. While the volume remains the same, the shape changes. Even the introduction of longitudinal and prognostic features for defining mental disorders (see p. 16) did not essentially change that reality. A new kind of conceptualisation began only after the pharmacological revolution in the middle of the twentieth century. The introduction of the new pharmacopsychiatry involving antipsychotics, antidepressants and mood stabilisers did not simply offer new modes of treatment, but also cleared the way for deeper and more fundamental consequences: they were social, ideological, methodological, conceptual, clinical, therapeutic and biological. The diagnosis and classification of mental disorder became more operationalised and standardised than in previous decades. Because of this, diagnosis in psychiatry became international and global, causing regional or national diagnostic concepts to gradually lose their importance. Diagnoses like 'schizophrenia' or 'affective disorders' were no longer 'private' or 'national' diagnoses. The separation, however, of the operationally defined schizophrenia from affective disorders left an undefined group of psychotic disorders belonging neither to schizophrenia, nor to affective disorders. Schizophrenia and affective disorders became more or less the sculptures, but other psychoses that were difficult to define remained the unformed and confused clay material left in the workshop of the sculptor – in this case, of the psychiatrist. Efforts to give even

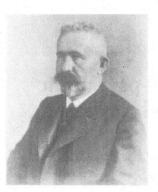

Fig. 1.1.   Emil Kraepelin (1856–1926): the Great Sculptor.

this material a form by naming it 'schizoaffective disorders' were only partially successful (Marneros and Tsuang, 1986; Marneros *et al.*, 1991b; Marneros, 1999, 2003; Marneros and Angst, 2000). Even after the creation of a smaller sculpture: 'schizoaffective disorders', some material remained undefined, confused and unnamed, but nevertheless unable to be ignored. It is present, which means that many people are suffering from some psychotic disorders that are not schizophrenia, that are not an affective disorder, and that are not a schizoaffective disorder, but something else. Since the beginning of scientific psychiatry, but especially after Kraepelin's dichotomous division of the so-called endogenous psychoses into schizophrenia (dementia praecox) and affective disorders (manic-depressive insanity), various concepts in many countries around the world have tried to define and describe this difficult part of the psychotic material: the non-schizophrenic, non-affective, non-schizoaffective, psychotic disorders (see Chapter 2).

One hundred years ago, Emil Kraepelin (Fig. 1.1) had the vision or the hope to have disease entities in psychiatry – as in the other domains of medicine. According to his principle, disease entities in psychiatry have to be determined by identical symptoms, identical course, identical aetiology, identical pathomorphology and identical treatment. Kraepelin's vision of disease entities still remains, however, only a dream of psychiatrists. Nevertheless, after the psychopharmacological revolution in psychiatry at the beginning of the 1950s, the speed of the psychiatric research aiming to achieve the goal defined by Kraepelin accelerated significantly. Biological research – including the biochemical and pathomorphological correlates demanded by Kraepelin – although still far from a conclusion, is also far from the beginning. Genetic research in psychiatry has been revitalised, partly as a result of the new operationalism following the pharmacopsychiatric revolution. But the fundamental condition for successful biological, pharmacological and genetic research, in other words, the *conditio sine qua non* for the realisation of Kraepelin's vision of nosological entities in psychiatry, is the reliable definition of syndromes and their homogeneous clustering or classification.

The modern positions: ICD-10 and DSM-IV definitions

The modern diagnostic systems such as the International Classification of Diseases (ICD-10; WHO, 1992) and the *Diagnostic and Statistical Manual* (DSM-IV, APA, 1994) recognise the area between schizophrenia, affective and schizoaffective disorders. They tried to homogenise the various regional and national concepts creating the group of 'Brief Psychoses' (DSM-IV) or 'Acute and Transient Psychotic Disorders' (ICD-10). Before we discuss the concepts leading to the definition of 'Brief Psychoses', as well as those leading to the definition of 'Acute and Transient Psychotic Disorders' (ATPD), we describe the modern definitions (DSM-IV and ICD-10).

DSM-IV definitions

DSM-IV defines the category of 'Brief Psychotic Disorder' (298.8). The essential feature of Brief Psychotic Disorder, according to DSM-IV, is a disturbance that involves *the sudden onset of delusions, hallucinations, disorganised speech or grossly disorganised or catatonic behaviour.* At least one of the psychotic symptoms has to be present. An episode of the disorder lasts *at least 1 day, but less than 1 month, and the individual eventually has a full return to the premorbid level of functioning* (see Table 1.1).

The DSM-IV recognises *three specifications* for Brief Psychotic Disorder based on the presence or absence of precipitating factors. To the diagnosis 'Brief Psychotic Disorder' can be added the specification 'With Marked Stressor(s)' if psychotic symptoms occur shortly after, and apparently in response to, one or more events that, singly or together, would be markedly stressful to almost anyone in similar circumstances in the person's culture. The subtype 'Brief Psychotic Disorder With Marked Stressor(s)' of DSM-IV is identical to the 'Brief Reactive Psychosis' of DSM-III-R. The problem of determining whether a specific stressor is a precipitant or a consequence of the psychotic disorder is recognised by DSM-IV. In such instances, the decision depends on factors such as the temporal relationship between the stressor and the onset of the symptoms, ancillary information from the spouse or friend about the level of functioning prior to the stressor, and the history of similar responses to stressful events in the past.

The specifier 'Without Marked Stressor(s)' may be noted if the psychotic symptoms do not occur shortly after, or are not apparently in response to, events that would be markedly stressful to almost anyone in similar circumstances in the person's culture.

Table 1.1. Diagnostic criteria for Brief Psychotic Disorder according to DSM-IV

A   Presence of one (or more) of the following symptoms:

- delusions
- hallucinations
- disorganised speech (e.g. frequent derailment or incoherence)
- grossly disorganised or catatonic behaviour

Note: Do not include a symptom if it is a culturally sanctioned response pattern.

B   Duration of an episode of the disturbance is at least 1 day but less than 1 month, with eventual full return to premorbid level of functioning.

C   The disturbance is not better accounted for by a Mood Disorder With Psychotic Features, Schizoaffective Disorder, or Schizophrenia and is not due to the direct physiological effects of a substance (e.g. a drug of abuse, a medication) or a general medical condition.

Specify if:

With Marked Stressor(s) (brief reactive psychosis): if symptoms occur shortly after and apparently in response to events that, singly or together, would be markedly stressful to almost anyone in similar circumstances in the person's culture

Without Marked Stressor(s): if psychotic symptoms do not occur shortly after, or are not apparently in response to events that, singly or together, would be markedly stressful to almost anyone in similar circumstances in the person's culture

With Postpartum Onset: if onset within 4 weeks postpartum

The third specifier 'With Postpartum Onset' may be noted if the onset of the psychotic symptoms is within 4 weeks postpartum. Apparently, DSM-IV recognised this specifier not only as an unspecific stressor, but also because of its possible etiological relevance (Lanczik *et al.*, 1990; Rohde and Marneros, 1992; Schöpf and Rust, 1994a,b).

The relation of 'Brief Psychotic Disorder' to cycloid psychosis (see p. 18) or to the bouffée délirante (see p. 24) is evident when we consider the 'associated features and disorders' listed in DSM-IV: individuals with Brief Psychotic Disorders typically experience emotional turmoil or overwhelming confusion. They may have rapid shifts from one intense affect to another. Although brief, the level of impairment may be severe, and supervision may be required to ensure that nutritional and hygienic needs are met and that the individual is protected from the consequences of poor judgement, cognitive impairment or acting on the basis of delusions. There appears to be an increased risk of mortality, with a particularly high risk of suicide, especially among younger individuals. Pre-existing personality disorders (e.g. paranoid, histrionic, narcissistic, schizotypal or borderline personality disorder) may predispose the individual to the development of the disorder.

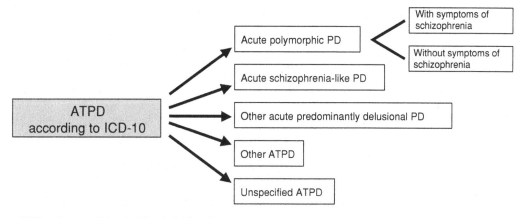

ATPD : Acute and Transient Psychotic Disorder
PD : Psychotic Disorder

Fig. 1.2.   Subtypes of ATPD (F23, ICD-10).

When making a diagnosis of 'Brief Psychotic Disorder', it is necessary to be aware of culturally sanctioned response patterns. In some religious ceremonies, for example, an individual may report hearing voices, but these do not generally persist and are not perceived as abnormal by most members of the person's community. Although this reference of DSM-IV is very important, it is nevertheless also problematic. The perception of hallucinations as not 'abnormal' by the members of a cultural community cannot always be a tip for the psychiatrist not to assume that they are indeed psychotic.

Brief Psychotic Disorder as defined by DSM-IV may appear in adolescence or early adulthood, with the average age at onset being in the late 20s or early 30s. By definition, a diagnosis of Brief Psychotic Disorder requires a full remission of all symptoms and a return to the premorbid level of functioning within 1 month of the onset of the disturbance. In some individuals, the duration of psychotic symptoms may be quite brief (e.g. a few days).

The Brief Psychoses in ICD-10

There is no definition of 'Brief Psychotic Disorder' in ICD-10, but there is an equivalent group – although more voluminous than in DSM-IV – namely, the 'Acute and Transient Psychotic Disorders' group (ATPD) (F23). The 'Acute and Transient Psychotic Disorders' group of ICD-10 is not only more voluminous than the 'Brief Psychotic Disorder' group of DSM-IV, but also much more differentiated. It is nominally divided into five subgroups, as shown in Fig. 1.2. However, the World Health Organization (WHO) points out that the present state of knowledge does not allow the reliable definition of this group and its subgroups. In the absence of a tried and tested multiaxial system, a diagnostic sequence was constructed that reflects the order of priority given to selected key features of the disorder (WHO, 1992).

The WHO requested that the features used for the definition of ATPD conform to the following order of priority:

1. acute onset within 2 weeks as the defining feature of the whole group
2. presence of typical syndromes
3. presence of acute stress.

Regarding 1:

Acute onset is defined as the change from a non-psychotic to a clearly psychotic state within 2 weeks or less. The distinction between 'abrupt' and 'acute' onset is recommended because there is some evidence that the prognosis of ATPD with abrupt onset could be more favourable (more than 48 hours, but less than 2 weeks).

Regarding 2:

Typical syndromes are firstly, the quickly changing and variable manifestations called 'polymorphic', and secondly, the presence or lack of typical schizophrenic symptoms.

Regarding 3:

The association with *acute stress* follows the tradition of the 'reactive' or 'psychogenic' psychoses (Strömgren, 1986). Nevertheless ATPD can be manifested without an association with acute stress; therefore making its presence not decisive for the diagnosis.

According to the WHO, a full remission can be achieved within 2 or 3 months, but often even after a few weeks or a few days. Nevertheless, some patients may develop persistent alterations. The present state of knowledge, however, does not allow for a definition of prognostic predictors.

Diagnostic criteria for the general category of ATPD can be found in Table 1.2. As with DSM-IV, the ICD-10 determines that the onset of the disorder occurs:

• '*with associated acute stress*' (the first psychotic symptoms occur within about 2 weeks of one or more events that would be regarded as stressful to most people in similar circumstances, within the culture of the person concerned)
• or '*without associated acute stress*'.

For research purposes, it is recommended that the change of the disorder from a non-psychotic to a clear psychotic state could be specified further as either:

• *abrupt* (onset within 48 hours) or
• *acute* (onset in more than 48 hours, but less than 2 weeks).

The definition of Acute and Transient Psychotic Disorders by the WHO aims to take into account various more or less national concepts, definitions and nomenclatures, as can be seen in Table 1.3. In the following paragraphs, the subgroups of Acute and Transient Psychotic Disorders are described.

Table 1.2. Acute and Transient Psychotic Disorders according to ICD-10 (F23)

G1	There is acute onset of delusions, hallucinations, incomprehensible or incoherent speech, or any combination of these. The time interval between the first appearance of any psychotic symptoms and the presentation of the fully developed disorder should not exceed 2 weeks.
G2	If transient states of perplexity, misidentification, or impairment of attention and concentration are present, they do not fulfil the criteria for organically caused clouding of consciousness as specified for F05, criterion A.
G3	The disorder does not meet the symptomatic criteria for manic episode (F30), depressive episode (F32), or recurrent depressive disorder (F33).
G4	There is insufficient evidence of recent psychoactive substance use to fulfil the criteria for intoxication (F1x.0), harmful use (F1x.1), dependence (F1x.2), or withdrawal states (F1x.3 and F1x.4). The continued moderate and largely unchanged use of alcohol or drugs in amounts or with the frequency to which the individual is accustomed does not necessarily rule out the use of F23; this must be decided by clinical judgement and requirements of the research project in question.
G5	Most commonly used exclusion clause. There must be no organic mental disorder (F00–F09) or serious metabolic disturbances affecting the central nervous system (this does not include childbirth). (The duration of the disorder must not exceed 3 months in subtypes F23.0, F23.3 and F23.8; it must not exceed 1 month in the subtypes F23.1 and F23.2, which include schizophrenic symptoms.)

Table 1.3. Synonyms for ATPD

- acute (undifferentiated) schizophrenia
- bouffée délirante
- cycloid psychoses
- oneirophrenia
- paranoid reaction
- psychogenic (paranoid) psychosis
- reactive psychosis
- schizophrenic reaction
- schizophreniform attack or psychosis
- remitting schizophrenia
- good prognosis schizophrenia

Acute Polymorphic Psychotic Disorder

Together, the first two subcategories of ATPD (F23.0 and F23.1) form the group of 'Acute Polymorphic Psychotic Disorder'. This group is *characterised by a rapidly changing and variable state (the 'polymorphic' state), in which symptoms change*

Table 1.4. Acute Polymorphic Psychotic Disorder Without Symptoms of Schizophrenia (F23.0)

A   The general criteria for acute and transient psychotic disorders (F23) must be met.

B   Symptoms change rapidly in both type and intensity from day to day or within the same day.

C   Any type of either hallucination or delusion occurs, for at least several hours, at any time from the onset of the disorder.

D   Symptoms from at least two of the following categories occur at the same time: emotional turmoil, characterised by intense feelings of happiness or ecstasy, or overwhelming anxiety or marked irritability; perplexity, or misidentification of people or places; increase or decreased motility, to a marked degree.

E   If any of the symptoms listed for schizophrenia (F20.0–F20.3), criterion G(1) and (2), are present, they are present only for a minority of the time from the onset, i.e. criterion B of F23.1 is not fulfilled.

F   The total duration of the disorder does not exceed 3 months.

Table 1.5. Acute Polymorphic Psychotic Disorder With Symptoms of Schizophrenia (F23.1)

A   Criteria A, B, C, and D of acute polymorphic psychotic disorder (F23.0) must be met.

B   Some of the symptoms for schizophrenia (F20.0–F20.3) must have been present for the majority of the time since the onset of the disorder, although the full criteria need not be met, i.e. at least one of the symptoms in criteria G1(1)a to G1(2)c.

C   The symptoms of schizophrenia in criterion B above do not persist for more than 1 month.

rapidly in both type and intensity from day to day or even within the same day.
Other features of Acute Polymorphic Psychotic Disorder are emotional turmoil, which may involve intense feelings of happiness or ecstasy, overwhelming anxiety or marked irritability, perplexity, the misidentification of people or places and markedly increased or decreased motility. The similarity to the 'cycloid disorder' (see p. 18) is obvious.

The Acute Polymorphic Psychotic Disorder is divided into a subtype '*without*' and a subtype '*with symptoms of schizophrenia*' (see Tables 1.4 and 1.5). Included in the group of 'Acute Polymorphic Psychotic Disorder with Symptoms of Schizophrenia' are – in addition to the features listed in Table 1.4 – some of the symptoms of schizophrenia, as listed in Table 1.6. The relation of Acute Polymorphic Psychotic Disorder *with* Symptoms of Schizophrenia to Acute Polymorphic Psychotic Disorder *without* Symptoms of Schizophrenia, and the question of whether there is any necessity for such a distinction, has been one of the topics of the Halle Study on Brief and Acute Psychoses (HASBAP). The discussion of this issue can be found on page 176.

Table 1.6. Schizophrenic symptoms according to ICD-10

(a)	thought echo, thought insertion or withdrawal, or thought broadcasting
(b)	delusions of control, influence, or passivity, clearly referred to body or limb movements or specific thoughts, actions, or sensations; delusional perception
(c)	hallucinatory voices giving a running commentary on the patient's behaviour, or discussing the patient among themselves, or other types of hallucinatory voices coming from some part of the body
(d)	persistent delusions of other kinds that are culturally inappropriate and completely impossible (e.g. being able to control the weather, or being in communication with aliens from another world)
(e)	persistent hallucinations in any modality, when occurring every day for at least 1 month, when accompanied by delusions (which may be fleeting or half-formed) without clear affective content, or when accompanied by persistent over-valued ideas
(f)	neologisms, breaks, or interpolations in the train of thought, resulting in incoherence or irrelevant speech
(g)	catatonic behaviour, such as excitement, posturing or waxy flexibility, negativism, mutism, and stupor.

Table 1.7. Acute Schizophrenia-like Psychotic Disorder (F23.2)

A	The general criteria for acute and transient psychotic disorders (F23) must be met.
B	The criteria for schizophrenia (F20.0–F20.3) are met, with the exception of the criterion for duration.
C	The disorder does not meet criteria B, C, and D for acute polymorphic psychotic disorder (F23.0).
D	The total duration of the disorder does not exceed 1 month.

Acute Schizophrenia-like Psychotic Disorder (ICD-10: F23.2)

For the diagnosis of *Acute Schizophrenia-like Psychotic Disorder*, in addition to the general criteria of ATPD, the criteria of schizophrenia must be fulfilled, with the exception of the criterion of time. Hence, this disorder distinguishes itself from schizophrenia mainly through the duration of the symptoms: if the total duration of the 'schizophrenic' symptoms is more than 1 month, then 'schizophrenia' should be diagnosed (Table 1.7). The relation of 'Acute Schizophrenia-like Psychotic Disorder' to 'Acute Polymorphic Disorder' is discussed, based on the findings of the HASBAP, on page 179.

Other Acute Predominantly Delusional Psychotic Disorders (F23.3)

The main features of these disorders are relatively stable delusions and/or hallucinations which do not fulfil the symptomatic criteria for schizophrenia (see Table 1.8).

The category 'Other Acute and Transient Psychotic Disorders' is to be diagnosed in patients with ATPD not belonging to the above-mentioned categories (Table 1.9).

Table 1.8. Other Acute Predominantly Delusional Psychotic Disorders (F23.3)

A   The general criteria for acute and transient psychotic disorders (F23) must be met.
B   Relatively stable delusions and/or hallucinations are present but do not fulfil the symptomatic criteria for schizophrenia (F20.0–F20.3).
C   The disorder does not meet the criteria for acute polymorphic psychotic disorder (F23.0).
D   The total duration of the disorder does not exceed 3 months.

Table 1.9. Other Acute and Transient Psychotic Disorders (F23.8)

Any other acute psychotic disorders that are not classifiable under any other category in F23 (such as acute psychotic states in which definite delusions or hallucinations occur but persist for only small proportions of the time) should be coded here. States of undifferentiated excitement should also be coded here if more detailed information about the patient's mental state is not available, provided that there is no evidence of an organic cause.

Table 1.10. Differences in definition between DSM-IV Brief Psychotic Disorder and ICD-10 Acute and Transient Psychotic Disorders

	Brief Psychotic Disorder	ATPD
Duration	1 day to 1 month	up to 3 months *exceptions* 'With Symptoms of Schizophrenia' and 'Acute Schizophrenia-like Psychotic Disorder' In these cases less than 1 month
Full development	Not specified	Less than 2 weeks
Symptoms	Any 'positive' symptom including disorganised speech and grossly disorganised behaviour	Any 'positive' symptom including incomprehensible or incoherent speech
		Polymorphic symptoms define subtype

Acute and Transient Psychotic Disorder, Unspecified (F23.9)

Acute and Transient Psychotic Disorder, Unspecified (F23.9) is the code for cases of ATPD without documented subclassification.

Differences in definition between the 'Brief Psychotic Disorder' of DSM-IV and that of 'Acute and Transient Psychotic Disorders' of ICD-10

The definition 'Brief Psychotic Disorder' of DSM-IV is not identical with that of 'Acute and Transient Psychotic Disorder' of ICD-10. The main points of difference between the two subgroups are listed in Table 1.10. The most crucial difference between the two definitions concerns the duration of the episode. While the duration of Brief Psychotic Disorder has to be at least 1 day, but not more than 1 month, the duration of ATPD could be extended up to 3 months. If schizophrenic symptoms are present (i.e. in the subgroups 'With Symptoms of Schizophrenia' and 'Acute Schizophrenia-like Psychotic Disorder'), the duration of ATPD must be less than 1 month.

The second main difference between the diagnostic categories of DSM-IV and ICD-10 concerns the time of the development of the full episode. For ATPD, an interval of up to 2 weeks is allowed between the first psychotic symptom and the fully developed disorder. There is no similar criterion for 'Brief Psychotic Disorder' in DSM-IV. Some differences between both psychotic disorders concern the symptomatology. DSM-IV demands the presence of one or more 'positive' symptoms, namely delusions, hallucinations, disorganised speech and grossly disorganised or catatonic behaviour. In ATPD, 'positive' psychotic symptoms also have to be present. In addition, a special 'polymorphic' syndrome serves to define the subgroup of Acute Polymorphic Psychotic Disorder. In the context of the HASBAP, the issue of concordance of ATPD and BP is discussed further in the following section.

Concordance of ICD-10 ATPD and DSM-IV BP

Concordance with DSM-IV diagnoses

By definition, patients fulfilling the DSM-IV BP criteria also fulfil the ICD-10 criteria for ATPD, but not those of other ICD-10 psychotic groups. *In other words: all DSM-IV (BP) patients are also ICD-10 ATPD*, but the same is not true vice versa.

In a study of Jørgensen and co-workers (1996) 17 of 51 patients with ATPD met the criteria of DSM-IV BP; the remaining patients were diagnosed as DSM-IV Schizophreniform Disorder or Psychotic Disorder Not Otherwise Specified. The Halle Study on Brief and Acute Psychoses (HASBAP) that is described in more detail below, investigated the diagnostic concordance of ATPD subtypes and DSM-IV categories by pairwise comparison of the respective subgroups using kappa statistics. There was a moderate, but significant concordance between a diagnosis of 'Schizophreniform Disorder' (295.40), according to DSM-IV, and the 'Schizophrenia-like' subtype of ATPD (F23.2), according to ICD-10 (kappa = 0.302, $P = 0.049$). Likewise, there was a significant concordance between the DSM-IV diagnosis 'Brief Psychosis' (298.8) and the ICD-10 diagnosis 'Acute Polymorphic Psychotic Disorder Without Symptoms of Schizophrenia' (F23.0) of ICD-10 (kappa = 0.294, $P = 0.025$). Significant concordance was also found for the delusional subgroups and the residual categories, although the numbers of patients in these subgroups were very small. The concordance values for all other pairs of diagnoses were non-significant or negative (Table 1.11) (see also Pillmann *et al.*, 2002).

Table 1.11. Concordance of ICD-10 ATPD and DSM-IV BP

	DSM-IV diagnosis			
ICD-10 diagnosis	Schizophreniform Disorder 295.40	Brief Psychotic Disorder 298.8	Psychotic Disorder NOS 298.9	Delusional Disorder 297.1
Acute Polymorphic Psychosis Without Symptoms of schizophrenia (F23.0)	−0.364*	0.294*	0.045	−0.047
Acute Polymorphic Psychosis With Symptoms of Schizophrenia (F23.1)	0.182	−0.059	−0.091	−0.047
Acute Schizophrenia-like Psychoses (F23.2)	0.302*	−0.155	−0.088	−0.046
Other Acute Predominantly Delusional Psychoses (F23.3)	−0.046	−0.048	−0.033	1.00***
Other Acute and Transient Psychoses (F23.8)	−0.090	−0.019	0.475***	−0.033

Cohen's kappa values given (*$P < 0.05$, ***$P < 0.001$).

Similarities and differences between ICD-10 ATPD and DSM-IV 'Brief Psychosis' patients

The 'Halle Study on Brief and Acute Psychoses' also addressed the question of similarities or differences between ATPD and DSM-IV BP patients. The sample was divided into two groups: 'Brief Psychotic Disorder' ($n = 26$) and 'Non-Brief Psychotic Disorder' ($n = 16$). Then the relevant characteristics were compared, such as gender, age at onset, number of episodes, course and outcome (Pillmann et al., 2002).

The main difference between DSM-IV BP and non-BP was found to be the longer duration of non-BP psychoses. This is a fact which goes without saying. This difference was evident both in terms of the duration of the psychotic period and in the length of hospitalisation. The longer duration of the non-BP subgroup, however, follows directly from the definition of ATPD and BP: of necessity, all ATPD lasting longer than 1 month have to be allocated to the non-BP category. There was also a significantly higher frequency of abrupt onset in BP. This difference, however, did not lead to a difference in outcome between BP and non-BP.

Except for duration of episode and mode of onset, *the two groups proved markedly similar*. This applied to sociodemographic features, gender distribution, age at onset, course and outcome, as measured by several indices of symptoms and general functioning (Pillmann *et al.*, 2002).

A *severe psychosocial stressor at onset of the disorder was rarely found* and thus seems not to be a prominent feature of BP. The rarity of relevant stressors before onset is an argument against an important pathogenetic role of psychogenic stress in this group of psychotic disorders as proposed by some theories of Acute Brief Psychoses (Dahl *et al.*, 1992; Okasha *et al.*, 1993; Ungvari and Mullen, 2000). Moreover, it confirms the decision of DSM-authors not to preserve the DSM-III-R category of Brief Reactive Psychosis – for which an acute stressor was mandatory – in DSM-IV.

It can be concluded *that DSM-IV BP shows considerable overlap with ICD-10 ATPD. Psychosocial stress proved not to be characteristic of BP, thus supporting the abandonment of the DSM-III-R concept of Brief Reactive Psychosis in DSM-IV. Most importantly, during long-term course, patients with ATPD do not fare worse than patients with BP. The relatively benign prognosis of BP therefore also extends to psychoses of a duration exceeding the maximum duration of 1 month demanded by DSM-IV.* This calls into question the strict 1-month duration criterion of BP in DSM-IV. Some authors have argued already for a longer duration criterion (Susser *et al.*, 1995b). Mojtabai and co-workers (2000), in a recent re-analysis of data from the WHO Determinants of Outcome of Severe Mental Disorder Study, found most cases of remitting psychoses with acute onset have a duration of 2–4 months. The strict criterion of duration implemented in the DSM-IV definition of BP seems not to serve to define a subgroup of especially favourable prognosis and should therefore be re-considered. The results of the comparison of BP and non-BP can be summarised as follows:

Conclusion: 'Brief Psychosis' of DSM-IV does not differ from other 'Acute and Transient Psychotic Disorders' as defined by ICD-10 in all essential parameters. There is no necessity to consider them as a separate diagnosis.

Considering the above-mentioned results, we decided to include all Brief Psychoses in the broader group of ATPD in the remaining chapters of this book. There is no clinical, practical or theoretical reason to separate them.

2

Concepts and synonyma

The dichotomy which shows the polymorphism

The existence of acute psychoses of short duration, often having intense or even dramatic symptomatology, but also full remission, has always been well known to clinicians and has been described by almost all important authors of the Pre-Kraepelinian period. Its relevance became still greater after Emil Kraepelin's division of the so-called endogenous or functional psychoses into a group of dementia praecox (i.e. schizophrenia) and manic-depressive insanity (mood disorders) (Kraepelin, 1893, 1896, 1899). Kraepelin based this dichotomy mainly on symptomatology, course and longitudinal outcome.

Mood disorders (i.e. manic-depressive insanity) are characterised according to Kraepelin by:
(a) severe depression or exaltation, or by a mixture of both (mixed states),
(b) a periodic or phasic course, and
(c) a favourable long-term outcome.
Kraepelin's dementia praecox is characterised by:
(a) mood incongruent delusions and hallucinations,
(b) disorganised behaviour,
(c) disturbances of volition, thinking or of affectivity,
(d) chronic and deteriorating course with an unfavourable outcome.
Kraepelin knew, of course, of Brief and Acute Psychoses: vivid descriptions of these disorders can be found in chapters on mixed states and, particularly, on delirious mania (Kraepelin, 1899/1990, see also below). Kraepelin allocated them according to the above-mentioned diagnostic criteria, especially the longitudinal prognostic criteria, either to manic-depressive insanity or to dementia praecox (i.e. schizophrenia). However, mainly because of their good prognosis, the vast majority of Brief and Acute Psychoses were allocated by Kraepelin and his fellows to the manic-depressive insanity group (Maj, 1984). An example of psychoses with acute polymorphic symptomatology, which according to the modern criteria would be

classified as Brief Psychotic Disorder or as Acute and Transient Psychotic Disorder, is the so-called 'delirious mania'. The typical picture of delirious mania has been described by Kraepelin in his textbook. The following passage is taken from the sixth edition, published in 1899, as translated into English by McQueen (Kraepelin, 1899/1990):

Another, rarer, form of manic excitement is characterised by the rapid development of deep, dreamlike clouding of the consciousness with numerous illusions and confused delusional ideas (delirious form). The attack usually begins very suddenly; only insomnia, restlessness or anxious depression may become noticeable a day or two or, more rarely, several weeks before-hand. The consciousness becomes clouded rapidly; the patients become seriously dazed, confused, mistake their surroundings and completely lose their orientation in time and space. Masses of illusions arise immediately. Everything is altered; it is burning; birds fly about in the air; angels appear; ghosts throw snakes in the patients' faces; shadows flit across the walls. They hear bells ringing, shooting, the sound of running water; the voice of God announces to them the Last Judgement, the redemption of all sins. The coffee smells of corpses, the hands are as if putrefied; the food tastes like goat's meat or human flesh, and the water tastes of sulphur. The head is all woozy, full of feverish heat; the patients believe themselves to be raised and to be cast into abysses; everything comes tumbling down around them. At the same time they develop muddleheaded, dreamlike delusional ideas. A terrible disaster is befalling them; the devil is coming; the patient must die, must go through dreadful struggles; he is poisoned, beheaded, is lost, damned, rotten, all alone in the world. Everything has been destroyed; his relatives have all died. He has won the jackpot, is proclaimed emperor, is the promised hero who is to save the world. The thousand-year Reich has dawned; the great battle with the Antichrist is being fought.

During this delirium the mood is very changeable, anxiously despondent ('thoughts of death') or whiningly fearful one moment, boisterously gay or exuberant or apathetic and indifferent the next. In the beginning, the patients often present the signs of the most senseless acute mania, chatter, shout, dance about, roll about on the ground, undress; they put up resistance, destroy things, empty their bowels and bladder beneath them, smear, make impulsive suicidal attempts and become recklessly violent. They are impossible to settle, give no information at all, pray, scold, beg for forgiveness; their incomprehensible, stammering utterances show extreme flight of ideas and distractibility. At times, they suddenly become quiet, but when this happens they are not lucid but incapable of gathering their thoughts together, confused, until the excitement begins again equally rapidly. There is usually almost complete sleeplessness during the first period. Food is frequently rejected; the nutrition declines very fast. The head quite often appears very flushed; the reflexes are lively; at times, distinct trembling is found all over the body, without any alcoholic basis.

The attack usually only remains at full pitch for a very short time. After a few days, or three to four weeks at the most, an abatement usually sets in quite rapidly. In some instances, all of the symptoms disappear from one day to the next; in most cases, though, this remission takes place more gradually. Single illusions, remains of the delusional ideas and particularly of the anomalies of mood remain for a little longer, after the excitement and confusion have already disappeared. The patients are at first still mistrustful, uncomprehending, discontented, irritable, probably also have some flight of ideas, especially in pieces of writing, are loquacious or unapproachable, feel an urge to go away, until by and by, in the course of a few weeks, even the last symptoms recede. The recollection of the delirious period is in most cases rather unclear; very often there is nearly total amnesia. (Kraepelin, 1899/1990)

It is evident that Kraepelin's description is largely identical to the ICD-10 description of 'Acute Polymorphic Psychotic Disorder'.

In addition, some patients allocated by Kraepelin (1899) to 'mixed states' fulfilled ICD-10 criteria for a 'Polymorphic Type of Acute and Transient Psychotic Disorder'. This is also the case with regard to the population of Kraepelin's pupil Wilhelm Weygandt, who wrote the first book in psychiatric literature on mixed states in 1899 (Weygandt, 1899; see also in Marneros and Angst, 2000; Angst and Marneros, 2001; Marneros, 2003).

Although Emil Kraepelin allocated all the 'functional' psychoses to 'dementia praecox' or 'manic-depressive insanity', he recognised that there is a 'not small group of disorders' which cannot be allocated – neither to schizophrenia, nor to affective disorders. He pointed out that such disorders could cause severe doubts regarding the reliability of his dichotomy (Kraepelin, 1920). Even after the reformation of Kraepelin's dichotomic system by Eugen Bleuler (1911) creating the 'group of schizophrenias', the problem of the brief, acute, transient and good prognosis psychoses has not been solved. In fact, all that was done was to move the category from Kraepelin's 'manic-depressive insanity' to Bleuler's 'schizophrenia'. A tradition which is still going on.

Opposition, especially in Germany, France, Scandinavia and Japan, to Emil Kraepelin's dichotomic system, as well as to Eugen Bleuler's conception of schizophrenia, formed very quickly. The main roots of the modern concepts of 'Acute and Transient Psychotic Disorders' given in the concepts of 'cycloid disorder' and 'bouffée délirante' can be found in Germany and France.

The cycloid psychoses

'Cycloid psychoses' is one of the main synonyms given by the WHO for 'Acute and Transient Psychotic Disorder'. The concept of cycloid psychoses is basic to the concept of 'Acute and Transient Psychotic Disorders', as well as to that of 'Brief Psychotic Disorder'. It was created and developed by the so-called , 'three Karls': Carl Wernicke, Karl Kleist and Karl Leonhard. The origin of cycloid psychoses can be found in the work of Carl Wernicke (Pillmann *et al.*, 2000a; Pillmann and Marneros, 2001), the concept and the name 'cycloid' in the work of his pupil Karl Kleist, and its completion in the work of Kleist's pupil, Karl Leonhard (see also Perris, 1986; Marneros, 1999; Sigmund and Mundt, 1999; Marneros and Angst, 2000; Beckmann and Franzek, 2001). The concept of the 'three Karls' focused mainly on clinical and,

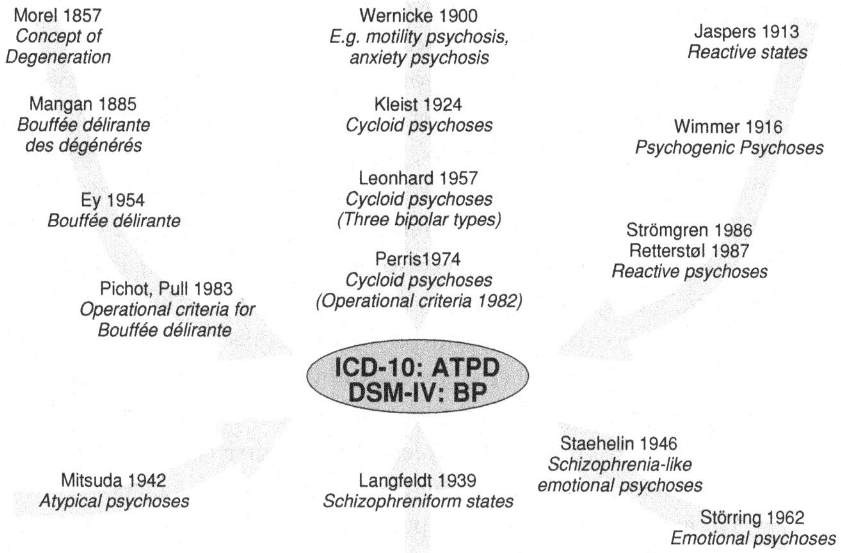

Morel 1857
Concept of
Degeneration

Wernicke 1900
E.g. motility psychosis,
anxiety psychosis

Jaspers 1913
Reactive states

Mangan 1885
Bouffée délirante
des dégénérés

Kleist 1924
Cycloid psychoses

Wimmer 1916
Psychogenic Psychoses

Ey 1954
Bouffée délirante

Leonhard 1957
Cycloid psychoses
(Three bipolar types)

Strömgren 1986
Retterstøl 1987
Reactive psychoses

Pichot, Pull 1983
Operational criteria for
Bouffée délirante

Perris 1974
Cycloid psychoses
(Operational criteria 1982)

ICD-10: ATPD
DSM-IV: BP

Staehelin 1946
Schizophrenia-like
emotional psychoses

Mitsuda 1942
Atypical psychoses

Langfeldt 1939
Schizophreniform states

Störring 1962
Emotional psychoses

Fig. 2.1.   Predecessors of ICD-10 Acute and Transient Psychotic Disorders and DSM-IV Brief Psychotic Disorder.

later, also on genetic findings (Neele, 1949; von Trostorff, 1968). The theoretical roots of the concept can be easily traced back to the work of Augustin Morel (1857) and to his concept of degeneration (see Fig. 2.1). Perris (1986) pointed out that it was very likely Valentin Magnan who linked an acute polymorphic psychotic disorder to a state of degeneration for the first time. In the 1880s, Magnan, inspired by Morel, described in some detail a psychopathological condition characterised by a sudden onset, a polymorphous symptomatology, and a recurrent course that was supposed to occur in successive generations of 'degenerate' families (see the next chapter on *bouffée délirante*). The idea of degeneration described a state of deviation from the norm that was mainly of hereditary origin and implied susceptibility for a number of disorders including 'degeneration psychosis'. The concept of 'degeneration psychosis' (later no longer linked to the hypothesis of 'degeneration') won acceptance in Germany and laid the foundation for the concept of 'cycloid psychoses'. Many important German authors of the first quarter of the twentieth century (e.g. Bonhoeffer, 1907; Schröder, 1918, 1920, 1922; Birnbaum, 1923, 1926; Binswanger, 1928) published important work on 'degenerative psychoses' (see Perris, 1986). Paul Schröder, who stressed the polymorphism of the picture of 'degenerative psychoses' (1920), was aware of the criticism against the concept of degeneration and wrote: '*albeit one should be more concerned with the essence of a problem rather than with its name, a bad name has a detrimental effect on the problem.*' He changed the term 'degenerative psychoses' into 'metabolic psychoses' (from the Greek verb *metaballein*, which translates to 'prone to change') to stress the polymorphism and the changeability of such psychotic disorders. But the term 'metabolic psychoses' has never caught on.

Carl Wernicke – German Professor of Psychiatry and Neurology in Breslau (today Wroclaw, Poland) and later at the University of Halle-Wittenberg – described the so-called, '*motility psychoses*', '*anxiety psychoses*' and '*expansive autopsychoses*' (Wernicke, 1900), which can be considered as the roots of cycloid disorders (Pillmann *et al.*, 2000a; Pillmann and Marneros, 2001). '*Motility psychoses*', as described by Wernicke, exist in two opposing forms, namely as 'hyperkinetic' and as 'akinetic' forms, which can also occur in combination. The dominant characteristic is a disturbance of motility with an increase or decrease in reactive and expressive moments and in 'pseudo-spontaneous movements'. In its akinetic form, the motility psychosis can be regarded as stupor and flexibilitas cerea. The fundamental symptom of '*anxiety psychoses*' (Wernicke, 1900) is anxiety with polymorphic fears, but also delusions, hallucinations and psychomotor disturbances.

Wernicke's most influential pupil was Karl Kleist (1879–1960), who was his co-worker in Halle-Wittenberg, and later Professor of Psychiatry in Rostock and Frankfurt/Main. Kleist coined the term 'cycloid psychoses', in 1924, and demanded a separation from Kraepelin's 'manic-depressive insanity'. Cycloid psychoses are, according to Kleist, bipolar disorders, but not belonging to the group of 'manic-depressive insanity', which is what we mean today by the term 'bipolar' (Kleist, 1924, 1925, 1926, 1928, 1953).

The first family study on cycloid psychoses was carried out in Karl Kleist's department by his pupil Edda Neele (1949). In her study on 'phasic psychoses', she distinguished between unipolar and bipolar disorders. Bipolar disorders included not only manic-depressive illness, but also the cycloid disorders. Neele maintained that cycloid disorders are clearly distinct from other forms of 'phasic psychoses' such as manic-depressive disease, and that each form is characterised by a homotypical family loading.

Karl Leonhard (1904–1988) completed the concept of cycloid psychoses. His most important aim was the identification of a great number of different psychotic disorders according to clinical, prognostic, and family characteristics. Leonhard created his 'classification of endogenous psychoses' as an independent and highly differentiated nosological system contrary to that of Kraepelin (Leonhard, 1957, English translation Leonhard, 1999). Leonhard allocated the cycloid psychoses into three pairs:
• the 'anxiety–happiness psychosis',
• the 'excited–inhibited confusion psychosis', and
• the 'hyperkinetic–akinetic motility psychosis'.
The three pairs of cycloid psychoses conceived by Leonhard were in accordance with Kleist's view that they were bipolar disorders (while differing essentially from manic-depressive illness) (Fig. 2.2).

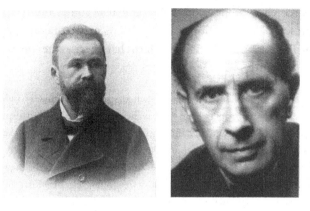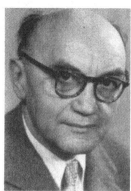

Carl Wernicke   Karl Kleist   Karl Leonhard

Fig. 2.2.   The three 'Karls': creators of the concept of cycloid psychoses.

The '*anxiety-happiness psychosis*' is characterised by a continuous change between severe all-pervasive anxiety and ecstatic happiness. It is possible that only one pole – anxiety or ecstasy – becomes manifest. Anxiety is often associated with delusions and hallucinations. While the experience of anxiety is overwhelming, its intensity fluctuates, and the patients can suddenly turn to a state of ecstatic happiness. In the happiness-ecstasy phase the patients experience a feeling of revelation and of closeness to God. They feel like wanting to help others, to save them, to make them as happy as they themselves are. A peculiarity of the affects of this condition is the character change during the episode. Clear-cut depressive or clear-cut manic mood is not recognisable or not long-lasting. An example given by Leonhard:

The patient 'became ill in 1934 after appendectomy and was admitted to the Frankfurt Hospital. He explained that the world had changed and was standing still. Simultaneously he had an elevated mood and he misjudged his environment. He thought a fellow patient was Hitler. Soon his mood became more anxious; he declared that the chimneys had stopped smoking and that it was probably his fault. Then an ecstatic phase followed during which he claimed that rays came from his hands, he had divine power, and he would establish a new religion. Periodically he developed incoherent pressure of speech. He sang, whistled, and made gymnastic movements. He spoke of angelic figures and of a spiritual face that he had seen. Although he seemed outwardly euphoric and laughed, he repeatedly spoke of a sin that he had committed. After eight weeks he calmed down and was discharged . . .'

The '*excited-inhibited confusion psychosis*' is characterised by thought disturbance, which in the excited type becomes incoherent accompanied by perplexity, but while in the inhibited pole, does not proceed forward. Incoherence is mostly manifest in an inconsistent choice of themes or by an inconsistent use of different languages.

In the most extremely inhibited form, the patient becomes mute. A wondering perplexity is present. Hallucinations and delusions are frequently present. Most often a polymorphous, rapidly changing pattern characterises the episodes of illness. An example of Leonhard:

'Mrs H., born in 1913, became ill in 1941. She was excited, spoke a lot, broke a window pane, and was admitted to the Frankfurt Hospital. Here she was cheerful, loquacious, and displayed flight of ideas. She misidentified people around her and confabulated that she had met the doctor 3 years earlier in a wine bar. Then her mood became more irritable, alternating between cheerfulness, irritability, and tearfulness. Her thought process became quite incoherent; for example, she said: 'I will also pull your feet – yes, a fallen woman – I love freedom – yesterday Kurt stood before the door, he had his heart in the right place – no, we don't need to die. . . .' She gave the doctor a false name and claimed he had an affair with her previously. She claimed that other people had several names and that a certain nurse was her biological sister. Frequently she scolded in a confused manner. After four months, the excitement receded and she was discharged. She calmed down at home and remained well.'

The main characteristic of the '*hyperkinetic–akinetic motility psychosis*' is a disturbance of motility. In the hyperkinetic type, there is an increase in reactive and expressive movements and in pseudo-spontaneous movements. In contrast to the increased activity of many patients, they do not suffer pressure of speech. The patients remain mute in the hyperkinetic phase. In the akinetic phase, only a few isolated movements are carried out. In extreme cases, the patient may lie completely motionless in stupor and in cataplexy. The difference to catatonia lies in the fact that the way in which movements are carried out is not qualitatively disordered in motility psychoses (Leonhard, 1961).

'Mrs. D., born in 1908, became ill in 1942. She was anxious, believing somebody wanted to poison her, and she was admitted to the Frankfurt Hospital. There she was perplexed, looked about anxiously, and asked, 'What am I accused of?' She distrusted her husband believing that he had incited other people against her, that he had been unfaithful, and that he wanted to get rid of her. She became increasingly restless, whined, jumped out of bed, ran around, wrung her hands, gesticulated continuously, held on to other patients, and climbed up on the window sill. After this excited condition had lasted three months suddenly she became akinetic. She was quite motionless, kept her eyes closed, had to be fed during which she barely opened her mouth; when she was brought to a sitting position she let her head fall forward. The phase continued four weeks, then excitement returned, which however stayed within moderate limits and gradually abated. She was well six months after admission, happy, lively, industrious, and could be discharged.'

According to Leonhard and his fellow researchers, patients with cycloid psychoses have a normal premorbid personality, are more frequently females, and become ill at the age of approximately 30 years. Forty per cent of patients show a family loading with 'endogenous psychoses' of the same type as those in the probands. The prognosis is always good (Leonhard, 1957; English transl. Leonhard, 1961, 1999). In many presentations during scientific meetings and also in personal discussions with the first author of this book, Leonhard pointed out that '*if the longitudinal prognosis is unfavourable, then you certainly made the false diagnosis "cycloid psychosis". You have to correct your diagnosis, even after many years*'.

In contrast to the reluctant response to Kleist's and Leonhard's general classification with its very subtle differentiation of 33 types of endogenous disorders, their special concept of cycloid psychoses found acceptance in several countries. Especially after the presentation of cycloid psychoses to the English-speaking countries by Fish (1964), they became known internationally. The main contributions to the internationalisation of the concept of cycloid psychoses were carried out by the Swedish psychiatrist Carlo Perris in co-operation with authors in other countries, such as Ian Brockington in Great Britain and Mario Maj in Italy (Mattsson and Perris, 1973; Perris, 1973, 1974, 1978, 1986; Perris and Perris, 1978; Perris *et al.*, 1979; Perris and Brockington, 1981; Brockington *et al.*, 1982a,b; Perris and Smigan, 1984; Maj, 1988, 1989, 1990a).

The 1974 study by Perris comprised a clinical and family investigation of 60 patients and their first- and second-degree relatives. The author recognised at the beginning of the study that a clear-cut distinction among the three different subtypes of cycloid psychoses proposed by Leonhard (1957) was not always possible. An admixture symptomatology of all three pairs of cycloid psychoses appeared to be more the rule than the exception. Perris did not find any convincing evidence that a differentiation into 'ideal' subtypes would have practical value. This knowledge led Perris (together with Brockington) to develop operational criteria for cycloid psychoses, ignoring Leonhard's differentiation of the three subgroups (Perris and Brockington 1981) (Table 2.1). The Perris studies verified the abrupt or acute onset of cycloid disorder: 'One of the investigated patients, who has been followed for several years and who has suffered several episodes, always becomes ill in the middle of the night after having gone to bed in a state of complete health' (Perris, 1974). Prodromal symptoms were found to be very rare, and when they occurred, they most often consisted of irritability and poor sleep. No seasonal dependence of onset was found. The development of psychotic symptoms was also very quick. They were mingled together without any discernible pattern and continuously changed, not only from day to day, but also in most instances from one hour to the next. The occurrence of schizophrenic first-rank symptoms (Schneider, 1959; Marneros, 1984) was very common. Further studies of Perris in co-operation with Brockington (Brockington *et al.*, 1982a,b) showed a very poor concordance between cycloid and schizoaffective psychoses. Only 20 of 108 patients who met the criteria of schizoaffective psychoses (mostly schizomanics) were diagnosed as cycloid.

Table 2.1. Diagnostic criteria for 'cycloid psychosis' (Perris and Brockington, 1981)

1. An acute psychotic condition, not related to the administration or the abuse of any drug or to brain injury, occurring for the first time in subjects in the age range 15–50 years.
2. The condition has a sudden onset with a rapid change from a state of health to a full-blown psychotic condition within a few hours or at most a very few days.
3. At least four of the following must be present:
   - confusion of some degree, mostly expressed as perplexity or puzzlement
   - mood-incongruent delusions of any kind: most often with a persecutory content
   - hallucinatory experiences of any kind, often related to themes of death
   - an overwhelming, frightening experience of anxiety, not bound to particular situations or circumstances (pananxiety)
   - deep feelings of happiness or ecstasy, most often with a religious colouring
   - motility disturbances of an akinetic or hyperkinetic type, which are mostly expressional
   - a particular concern with death
   - mood swings in the background and not so pronounced to justify a diagnosis of affective disorder.
4. There is no fixed symptomatological combination; on the contrary, the symptomatology may change frequently during the episode and shows a bipolar characteristic.

Patients identified as cycloid showed a significantly better short-term and long-term outcome than other psychotic patients did. Although the knowledge about epidemiology of cycloid psychotic disorder is still scanty, Perris assumed that 10–15% of psychotic patients are cycloid.

In Germany, there is still some research in the field of cycloid psychoses being performed mainly at the University of Würzburg (Beckmann *et al.*, 1990; Beckmann and Franzek, 2001, Franzek and Beckmann 1992, 1998a; Franzek *et al.*, 1996; Stöber *et al.*, 1997; Strik *et al.*, 1997). The work of the Würzburg group can be characterised as very close to the original concept of Leonhard. These authors reject the criteria of Perris and Brockington with the argument that the three sub-groups of cycloid psychoses are none the less clearly distinguishable. They carried out clinical, prognostic, family, twin, paraclinical and biological investigations in order to validate the concept of cycloid psychoses (Lanczik *et al.*, 1990; Beckmann *et al.*, 1990; Franzek and Beckmann 1992, 1998a; Strik *et al.*, 1993, 1997; Franzek *et al.*, 1996; Stöber *et al.*, 1997; Pfuhlmann *et al.*, 1998, 1999).

Bouffée délirante

'Bouffée délirante' is another important synonym given by the WHO for 'Acute and Transient Psychotic Disorders'. It can be regarded as the French root of ATPD

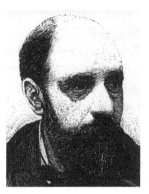

Fig. 2.3.   Valentin Magnan (1835–1916): the creator of the bouffée délirante.

and Brief Psychoses. The modern concept of bouffée délirante of Francophonic Psychiatry is based on operational criteria including a sudden onset, a specific symptomatology and the evolution of the disorder (Pichot, 1986a; Pull *et al.*, 1983).

The concept of the 'bouffée délirante' has been influential in French psychiatry for more than one hundred years (Appia, 1964; Pichot, 1986a, 1986b). As previously mentioned, in the 1880s Valentin Magnan (1835–1916) (Fig. 2.3) described for the first time a psychopathological condition, named '*syndromes épisodiques des dégénérés*' or '*bouffée délirante des dégénérés*'. The concept created by Magnan was completed by his pupils , Legrain and Saury (Legrain, 1886; Saury, 1886; Magnan and Legrain, 1895). It was later renewed by Henri Ey (1952, 1954). Magnan, the 'grey eminence' of French psychiatry (Shorter, 1997) and one of the most important French nosologists, worked at the Paris mental hospital Sainte-Anne. He was devoted to the study and propagation of the idea of 'degeneration', which had been introduced by Bénédict-Augustin Morel in 1857. The concept of degeneration combined three assumptions: the assumption that the liability to a number of psychiatric disorders and deficits is hereditary, the assumption that this liability is indicated by observable somatic and psychological abnormalities (the degenerate 'stigmata') and the assumption that the illnesses involved get worse as they are passed from generation to generation. Magnan extensively described the psychiatric disorders of the hereditary degenerates. He differentiated different grades of degeneration (including the 'dégénérés superieurs' of normal intelligence) and described in detail the degenerate stigmata. Particular stress was put by Magnan on the occurrence of specific psychotic illnesses of the degenerate that have been described in a differentiated way in the thesis of his pupil M. Legrain 'Du délire chez les dégénérés' (1886). Often these disorders take the form of psychotic disorders of acute onset and rapid remission, termed 'délire d'emblée' (sudden madness) or 'bouffées subites d'idées délirantes' (Legrain, 1886).

The clinical characteristics of bouffée délirante as given by Pichot (1986a) can be summarised as follows:

1. A sudden onset: 'Like a bolt from the blue, full-blown delusions suddenly shatter the poise of a fully rational mind . . . and flare up without premonitory signs.'

2. The symptomatology: 'The delusions are ripe from the onset . . . There is no warning sign. The delusions form and lurk fully developed in the mind, then burst forth with overpowering force, but fail to evolve further.' The delusional themes are numerous, diverse, and protean. The delusions are a loose, motley jumble, without recognisable structure and cohesiveness. They may be accompanied by hallucinations, but these are not an essential nor even constant feature. Combined with the delusions eventually some degree of confusion exists with affective symptoms of various types described by Legrain as ranging from anxiety, agitation, impulsiveness, and expansiveness to inertia.

3. The evolution: Normally there is no precipitating factor, or at most, minimal identifiable stress. The physical health of the patient is normal and remains so during the episode. A rapid return to the premorbid personality level is an essential diagnostic criterion (the French term *bouffée* – flare-up or outburst – implies suddenness of both onset and resolution). 'By definition, transitory delusional states are short-lived.' Relapses may, however, occur but, when occurring, are 'separated by symptom-free intervals.' Magnan speaks in these cases of 'recurrent transitory delusional states' (*bouffées délirantes à type intermittent*) (Pichot, 1986b).

From the nosological point of view, the 'polymorphous psychoses of the degenerates' were demarcated clearly from another important nosological entity in Magnan's psychiatry: the 'chronic psychotic disorder of systematic evolution' ('délire chronique à évolution systématique'), a disorder of systematic course leading to dementia. While the static nature of the status of a degenerate (the process of degeneration occurs across generations, not in the individual) explains the transient nature of the psychoses, Magnan was left with the problem that many patients suffering from the 'psychoses of the degenerates' did not display the signs of a severe state of degeneration (such as debility). Here the notion of the 'superior degenerate' was of help, denoting a subject in which degeneration is present despite seemingly intact intellectual functions. In these individuals, psychosis manifests itself through the imbalance of nervous centres, some irritated and some weakened.

Tragically, at the end of Magnan's life, his influence drastically diminished. Early in the twentieth century, many of Magnan's ideas, including the concept of bouffée délirante, had largely been abandoned. The theory of degeneration was strongly criticised (Shorter, 1997). In issues of classification, French psychiatry for some time was influenced largely by the new doctrine of Emil Kraepelin (Appia, 1964). It was Henri Ey who renewed interest in the entity of bouffée délirante which he

Table 2.2. Diagnostic criteria for 'bouffée délirante' (Pull et al., 1983)

1. Age of onset: approximately 20–40 years.
2. Onset: acute, without any prior psychiatric history (other than identical episodes).
3. No chronicity: active phases fade away completely in several weeks or months possibly recurring under the same form: the patient remaining devoid of all abnormality in the interval.
4. Characteristic symptoms (all of the following):
   Delusions and/or hallucinations of any type
   Depersonalisation/derealisation and/or confusion
   Depression and/or elation
   Symptoms vary from day to day even from hour to hour.
5. Not due to any organic mental disorder, alcoholism or drug abuse.

refined and contrasted to a more narrowly defined concept of schizophrenia (Ey, 1954). Its characteristics included, just as described by Magnan, a sudden onset and full remission, rapidly changing delusions and disturbance of consciousness. However, in his 'organo-dynamic' psychiatry, Ey was sceptical about static nosological entities (Ey, 1952). Instead, by means of a structural psychological analysis of the individual symptoms, he identified different levels of 'destructuration of consciousness'. In this theoretical framework, the bouffée délirante, among other acute psychoses, displays a level of destructuration intermediate to manic-depressive illness and schizophrenia. Hallmarks of this intermediate level of psychopathological disturbance are oneroid phenomena (Ey, 1954). It is this intermediate level of disturbance that explains the benign prognosis of the bouffée délirante. The diagnosis conforms with the desire of many French psychiatrists to put more weight on course than on symptomatology and to separate the acute psychoses from schizophrenia (Pull et al., 1984). Hence, the French psychiatric school even after the incorporation into its nosology of the Kraepelinan *dementia praecox* and later of the Bleulerian schizophrenia, has retained the category *bouffée délirante* as an independent mental disorder (Pichot, 1982). Bouffée délirante has its place in French psychiatry as documented by its inclusion in the national classification system INSERM (1969) and the formulation of operational criteria by Pull and co-workers (Pull et al., 1984, 1987) and the continuing publication of case reports, theoretical articles and clinical studies. The term, however, is not always used very strictly by French psychiatrists, e.g. it has also been applied to substance induced delirious states (Devillières et al., 1996).

The operational criteria of bouffée délirante that have been developed by Pull and his colleagues (1983) are shown in Table 2.2. Studies on bouffée délirante are mainly counfined to the French-speaking world with the exception of some polydiagnostic studies (Maj, 1989, 1990a; Copolov *et al.*, 1990). Ferrey and Zebdi (1999) investigated a clinical population and supported the assumption that bouffée délirante is not identical with schizophrenia. The better prognosis of bouffée délirante compared to schizophrenia could be confirmed in follow-up studies (Singer *et al.*, 1986; Lazaratou *et al.*, 1989), but not the stability of the diagnosis. Long-term studies showed subsequent diagnostic change to schizophrenia in 36% (Lazaratou *et al.*, 1989) and to 42% (Singer *et al.*, 1986) of cases initially diagnosed as bouffée délirante. Allodi (1982) tried to establish the concept of bouffée délirante in Canada. In developing countries, especially Francophone countries in Africa, the concept of bouffée délirante is also used (Collomb, 1965; Constant, 1972; Devillières *et al.*, 1996; Rouchouse, 1996). Ngoma and Mbungu (2000) published a study describing 121 cases with bouffée délirante in Kinshasa.

'Atypical psychoses' or 'Mitsuda psychoses'

Another synonym given by the WHO for 'Acute and Transient Psychotic Disorder' is that of 'atypical psychoses', which is mainly a Japanese concept (see Perris, 1986). The impact of German psychiatry has been noticeable in Japan, where the hypotheses of Kleist and Leonhard have been integrated in the genetic research by Mitsuda (1965), Mitsuda and Fukuda (1974), Kurosawa (1961) and in more comprehensive biological investigations by Hatotani and colleagues (Hatotani and Nomura, 1983; Hatotani, 1996).

The creator of the concept of 'atypical psychoses' in Japan was Hisatoshi Mitsuda, who presented the topic for the first time in 1941 therefore the name 'Mitsuda Psychoses'. The term 'atypical psychoses' is a term which has also been often used by Kleist and Leonhard (Leonhard, 1934, 1939). In contrast to Kleist and especially to Leonhard, Mitsuda had doubts regarding the full remission of all cases with 'atypical psychoses' (Mitsuda, 1965, Kimura *et al.*, 1984; overview in Fukuda, 1990). A national symposium took place in Japan in 1960 on 'atypical psychoses', which contributed to the establishment of the term in Japan. Hatotani (1983) described the basic clinical characteristics of 'atypical psychoses' as shown in Table 2.3. According to family studies by Mitsuda and Fukuda (1974), atypical psychoses have to be regarded as separate from both schizophrenia and depressive psychoses and from the epileptic psychoses, although some overlaps may occur. The case reports given by Kurosawa (1961), in a clinical and genetic study, contain descriptions that show marked similarities to the concept of cycloid psychoses. Some of Kurosawa's patients would be classified as typical cases of 'excited-inhibited confusion psychosis' or 'anxiety-happiness psychosis' according to Leonhard (Kurosawa, 1961). Mitsuda and Fukuda (1974) stressed that the pathology of 'typical' schizophrenia is that of

Table 2.3. Clinical characteristics of 'atypical psychoses' according to Hatotani (1983)

1. Acute onset of the illness.
2. Favourable prognosis.
3. Tendency toward relapse.
4. The basic mental symptoms are emotional disturbances, psychomotor disturbances and alterations of consciousness.
5. The emotional and psychomotor disturbances tend to alternate between extremes, such as manic depressive, anguished-ecstatic and excited-stuporous.
6. The premorbid personality of the patients in this group, in sharp contrast to more typical schizophrenics, is reality oriented and they have good affective rapport.

the personality, whereas the pathology of the 'atypical psychoses' is a pathology of consciousness, underlining their relationship with 'bouffée délirante' and the 'confusional cycloid psychoses'. It has been assumed that 'atypical psychoses' as defined by the Japanese psychiatrists have some similarities to epileptic psychoses. This assumption could not be supported in the HASBAP (Röttig, 2001) (see also p. 167ff).

The term 'atypical psychoses' has not only been used by Japanese psychiatrists, but also by many authors to characterise various conditions not fitting the classical Kraepelinian dichotomy (Pauleikhoff, 1969; Cerrolaza and Leghorn, 1971; Manschreck and Petri, 1978; Roth and McClelland, 1979; Remington *et al.*, 1990). In DSM-III and DSM-III-R, 'atypical psychoses' was also used as a synonym for the residual category of Psychotic Disorders Not Otherwise Specified (298.9). This category includes patients with psychotic symptomatology (i.e. delusions, hallucinations, disorganised speech, grossly disorganised or catatonic behaviour) not fulfilling the criteria for any specific psychotic disorder. Examples are postpartum psychoses not fulfilling the criteria of any other psychotic or organic disorder, psychoses failing to meet the duration criteria of a specific disorder and psychoses with unclear or unusual clinical symptoms that cannot be classified elsewhere. From these descriptions it becomes clear that the category 'Psychotic Disorders Not Otherwise Specified' in the DSM is a true 'residual' category and does not define a nosological entity. Consequently, in DSM-IV, the term 'atypical psychosis' is no longer mentioned as a synonym for this category.

'Reactive' or 'psychogenic' psychoses

'Reactive' or 'psychogenic' psychoses are also among the synonyms given by the WHO for 'Acute and Transient Psychotic Disorders'. So-called reactive/psychogenic psychoses have a very strong tradition mainly in Scandinavia (Strömgren, 1986) although the basic concept was developed by Karl Jaspers (Jaspers, 1913). The first monograph on the psychogenic psychoses was written by August Wimmer, who was Professor of Psychiatry at the University of Copenhagen from 1921 to 1937. His book was published in 1916 and represented the first comprehensive survey of the field (see also Strömgren, 1986). He wrote:

As psychogenic psychoses we designate … the various, clinically independent psychoses, the main feature of which is, that they – usually on a (definite) predisposed foundation – are caused by mental agents ('mental traumata'), and in such a way that these pathemata determine the point in time of the start of the psychosis, the fluctuations (remissions, intermissions, exacerbations) of the disease, very often also its cessation. Likewise the form and the content of the psychosis are, more or less directly and completely ('comprehensibly') determined by the precipitating mental factors. To these criteria can, finally, be added the predominant tendency of these disorders to recovery and, more specifically, that they never end in deterioration. (Translated by Strömgren 1986)

The concept of 'reactive' or 'psychogenic psychoses' developed by Wimmer is based on Jaspers' '*General Psychopathology*', in which he wrote in 1913:

Let us once more summarise the factors common to all genuine reactions: There is a precipitating factor, which stands in a close time relationship with the reactive state and has to be one which we can accept as adequate. There is a meaningful connection between the contents of the experience and those of the abnormal reaction. As we are concerned with a reaction to an experience, any abnormality will lapse with the course of time. In particular, the abnormal reaction comes to an end when the primary cause for the reaction is removed. Reactive abnormalities are therefore a complete contrast to all morbid processes which appear spontaneously.

Jaspers stressed that reactive states can be classified in different ways:
(a) according to what precipitates the reaction. As examples of precipitating factors, Jaspers mentioned those responsible for prison psychoses, for psychoses due to earthquakes and catastrophes, for reactions of homesickness, combat psychoses and psychoses of isolation, whether due to linguistic barriers or deafness.
(b) according to the particular psychic structure of the reactive states. Jaspers mentioned as possible types of psychic structure of the reactive states the ones listed in Table 2.4.
(c) according to the type of psychic constitution that determines the reactivity. Jaspers believed the majority of reactive states occur in people who have some kind of persistent, or transient, increased reactivity. However, some massive events can create short-lasting psychotic reactions even in quite normal people.
One should bear the latter point in mind (see also Strömgren, 1986).

Table 2.4. 'Reactive states' according to Jaspers (1913)

- Psychasthenic reactions, reactive depression.
- Impulsive reactions, fits, tantrums, rages, acts of violence, etc.; a working-up of the self into a state of narrowed consciousness, 'primitive reactions'.
- Syndromes with clouding of consciousness.
- Puerilism, hysterical delirium, stuporous pictures, ideas of persecution.
- Syndromes with hallucinations and delusions, acute paranoid reaction.

Table 2.5. Reactive (psychogenic) psychoses (according to Strömgren, 1986)

1. Emotional syndromes
   - Depressions
   - Excitations
   - Emotional paralysis.
2. Syndromes with disturbance of consciousness
   - Delirious states
   - Dissociative states, twilight states, fugues.
3. Paranoid (delusional) states
   - Sensitive delusions of reference
   - Litigious paranoia
   - Incarceration psychoses
   - Delusional psychoses in the deaf
   - Delusional psychoses in other forms of sensory deprivation
   - Psychoses following linguistic isolation
   - Induced psychoses.

Strömgren classified the 'reactive'/'psychogenic psychoses' as listed in Table 2.5.

In the third edition of the DSM, there was an attempt to give operational criteria for an entity called 'Brief Reactive Psychosis'. This condition was characterised by a sudden display of psychotic behaviour that lasts at least several hours, but less than 1 week. An acute and severe stressful event as a trigger was mandatory, such as the death of a loved one. In DSM-III-R the maximum duration of Brief Reactive Psychosis was changed to 1 month. Table 2.6 gives inclusion and exclusion criteria for Brief Reactive Psychosis according to DSM-III-R. Although the maximum duration has now been extended to 1 month, the definition is still rather restrictive when compared to the broader Scandinavian concept of reactive psychosis: strict criteria are set for duration, character of symptoms, and, in particular, for the severity of the mandatory stressor. Accordingly, Brief Reactive Psychosis proved to be a very rare condition, even among high risk groups such as Air Force recruits (Jauch and

Table 2.6. Defining criteria of Brief Reactive Psychosis according to DSM-III-R (APA, 1987)

A At least one of the following symptoms indicating impaired reality testing (not culturally sanctioned):

(1) incoherence or marked loosening of associations

(2) delusions

(3) hallucinations

(4) catatonic or disorganised behaviour.

B Emotional turmoil, i.e. rapid shifts from one intense affect to another, or overwhelming perplexity or confusion.

C Appearance of the symptoms in A and B shortly after, and apparently in response to, one or more events that, singly or together, would be markedly stressful to almost anyone in similar circumstances in the person's culture.

D Absence of the prodromal symptoms of Schizophrenia, and failure to meet the criteria for Schizotypical Personality Disorder before the onset of the disturbance.

E Duration of an episode of the disturbance of from a few hours to 1 month, with eventual full return to premorbid level of functioning. (When the diagnosis must be made without waiting for the expected recovery, it should be qualified as 'provisional'.)

F Not due to a psychotic Mood Disorder (i.e. no full mood syndrome is present), and it cannot be established that an organic factor initiated and maintained the disturbance.

Carpenter, 1988a,b; Beighley *et al.*, 1992). The concept has therefore been dropped from DSM-IV. In the category of Brief Psychotic Disorder of DSM-IV, the criterion of a severe stressor has been moved from a defining criterion to an optional specifier (see p. 5).

The original 'broad' concept of reactive psychoses is still being used in Scandinavia, where up to 13–30% of all psychiatric admissions are diagnosed with reactive psychosis (Dahl, 1986; Opjordsmoen, 2001). The concept has been strongly advocated by Strömgren (1986, 1987). More recently, Ungvari pleaded for the acceptance of an independent category 'reactive psychoses' (Ungvari *et al.*, 2000; Ungvari and Mullen, 2000).

Although according to WHO, the 'Reactive Psychoses' could be a synonym for ATPD, this is only true for a very small part of them. *Reactive psychoses differ from ATPD, mainly due to the criterion 'psychosocial precipitant', which must be present in reactive psychoses, but not in ATPD. Another significant difference from ATPD is the broad and unspecific constellation of symptoms of the 'reactive/psychogenic psychoses',* at least as presently diagnosed in Scandinavia. The symptoms include depressive, dissociative and other non-psychotic states (Table 2.5). Finally, the validation of the concept of reactive psychoses should still be regarded as poor (Jauch and Carpenter, 1988a,b).

Table 2.7. Defining criteria of Schizophreniform
Disorder according to Langfeldt (1939)

A Acute onset often in relation to a precipitating factor.
B Presence of confusion during the acute episode.
C Absence of schizoid personality traits.
D A pycnic body constitution.

'Schizophreniform disorder' and similar concepts

The concepts described above, namely cycloid psychoses, bouffée délirante, reactive/psychogenic psychoses and atypical psychoses, represent the most important attempts to delineate a group of acute and transient psychoses from schizophrenia and affective disorders. Many other attempts have also been carried out, which, however, show many similarities to the above-mentioned concepts.

'Dreamlike states', independent of organic conditions and not identical with schizophrenia, have been described by Mayer-Gross (1924) in Germany. The 'schizophrenia-like emotional psychoses', were described by Staehelin (1931, 1946) and Labhardt (1963) in Switzerland, and the 'emotional psychoses' by Störring and by his pupil Boeters in Germany (Störring *et al.*, 1962; Störring, 1969; Boeters, 1971). Psychiatrists in Spain, Portugal, Italy, Greece, Hungary, Bulgaria and Russia described states very similar to those mentioned above (overview in Perris, 1986). They shared clinical and prognostic features with the above-described disorders.

A very interesting contribution was that of the Norwegian psychiatrist Langfeldt. After the introduction of physical treatment methods (electroconvulsive therapy, insulin and cardiazol therapy) in the 1940s, it was observed that some cases of 'schizophrenia' respond favourably to such treatments while others fail to show a favourable response. Langfeldt (1939) assumed that the conflicting treatment results were caused by the inhomogeneity of what was called 'schizophrenia'. He attempted to differentiate between a nuclear group of schizophrenia with poor prognosis and a group of 'schizophreniform psychoses' with a much better spontaneous prognosis. The defining criteria of schizophreniform disorder according to Langfeldt are listed in Table 2.7. Some of Langfeldt's ideas are involved in modern diagnostic systems such as DSM-IV and ICD-10, although the concepts of Schizophreniform Disorders or Schizophrenia-like Psychoses of these two systems are different to those of Langfeldt (see p. 11 and Table 2.8). From Table 2.8 it becomes clear that *the main difference between DSM-IV schizophreniform disorder and DSM-IV schizophrenia concerns the 6-month duration criterion.* 'Good Prognostic Features' are only included as specifiers, but are not obligatory for diagnosis. Some authors have therefore argued that schizophreniform disorder is a heterogeneous category and that many patients with schizophreniform disorder would meet the full criteria

Table 2.8. Defining criteria of Schizophreniform Disorder according to DSM-IV

A Criteria A, D, and E of schizophrenia are met.[a]
B An episode of the disorder (including prodromal, active, and residual phases) lasts at least 1
  month but less than 6 months. (When the diagnosis must be made without waiting for
  recovery, it should be qualified as 'Provisional'.)
  Specify if:
  Without Good Prognostic Features
  With Good Prognostic Features: as evidenced by two (or more) of the following:
  (1) Onset of prominent psychotic symptoms
  (2) Confusion or perplexity at the height of the psychotic episode
  (3) Good premorbid social and occupational functioning
  (4) Absence of blunted or flat affect.

[a] These criteria include the presence of the characteristic symptoms of schizophrenia, the exclusion
of schizoaffective and mood disorders, and the exclusion of the effects of a substance or a general
medical condition causing the disorder.

for schizophrenia at a later time (Strakowski, 1994; Zhang-Wong *et al.*, 1995). In his
1994 review, Strakowski questioned the validity of a diagnosis of schizophreniform
disorder (Strakowski, 1994). Some authors have indeed found frequent diagnostic change to schizophrenia 2 years after the index episode (Zarate *et al.*, 2000).
The authors concluded that the diagnosis of schizophreniform disorder has no
value and should be discarded. Others have found evidence of a more favourable
outcome in schizophreniform disorder (Möller *et al.*, 1989; Zhang-Wong *et al.*,
1995).

The development in the USA was described in reviews by Vaillant (1964), Maj
(1984), Perris (1986) and Pichot (1986a). It can be assumed, according to these
authors, that one of the earliest papers on the topic was published by Kirby (1913).
On the basis of case reports, Kirby adopted the view that the occurrence of catatonic
symptoms was not only a phenomenon of dementia praecox, but could also be found
in cases of recurrent psychoses with a syndrome shift to manic-depressive episodes
during course. Acute onset and a precipitating stressful event were characteristics
of the patients described by Kirby.

Hoch (1921) described similar cases under the name 'benign stupor'. He assumed
that such cases were a new type of manic-depressive reaction. Some of Hoch's
patients were followed up by Rachlin (1935), who showed that most of them had
turned into deteriorated schizophrenia.

The 'schizo-affective psychoses' described by Kasanin (1933) in the USA also
belong to the efforts of limiting the concept of schizophrenia (see below). Vaillant
(1964) described 'Good Prognosis Schizophrenia', which also included Kasanin's

schizoaffective psychoses. Hunt and Appel (1936) described patients with characteristics of both schizophrenia and manic-depressive disorder, and were not very
happy that in the USA such 'hybrid nosological orphans' were usually forced into
a diagnosis of either schizophrenia or manic-depressive psychosis. The concept of
cycloid psychoses was known in the USA, but it seems that American authors understand the concept of cycloid psychoses as interchangeable with that of schizoaffective
psychoses (Procci, 1976; Grossman *et al.*, 1984; Perris, 1986).

The schizoaffective disorders

For a long time, schizoaffective disorders have been a controversially discussed, but
certainly existent, nosological category. Nevertheless, they are still an insufficiently
investigated area (overview in Marneros and Tsuang, 1986, 1990; Marneros *et al.*,
1991b; Marneros, 1999, 2003; Marneros and Angst, 2000). Long before the name
'schizoaffective' was used by John Kasanin in 1933 in the USA, the disorders referred
to by that name had already been described in Europe. Karl Kahlbaum is considered
the first psychiatrist of the modern era who placed schizoaffective disorders into a
separate group, which he called 'vesania typica circularis' (Kahlbaum, 1863). For
his definition, Kahlbaum applied cross-sectional and longitudinal aspects. Emil
Kraepelin also knew cases between 'Dementia Praecox' and 'Manic-Depressive
Insanity' (Kraepelin, 1920, 1896, 1893, 1899/1990). These 'cases-in-between' were
problematic for him because they contradicted his dichotomy of 'Dementia Praecox' and 'Manic-Depressive Insanity' (see p. 3ff). Kraepelin was always aware that
not all cases of 'endogenous' mental disorders could be classified without difficulties
into the two categories. In a paper he wrote in 1920 entitled 'Die Erscheinungsformen des Irreseins' (manifestations of insanity), which was cited above, he admitted
that the boundaries between the two major groups of mental disorders were very
elastic and that there were 'many overlaps (between schizophrenia and affective
disorders) in this area' (Kraepelin, 1920).

Eugen and Manfred Bleuler (1911, 1972) knew of and described such overlaps
and named them 'Mischpsychosen' (mixed psychoses). They allocated the 'mixed
psychoses' to schizophrenia because of the primacy they gave to the so-called 'fundamental symptoms'. According to Bleuler's concept, only the presence of fundamental
symptoms was decisive for the diagnosis of schizophrenia; not the course nor the
outcome. Only in 1966 did the scholar and fellow of Manfred Bleuler, Jules Angst,
investigate 'mixed psychoses' as a part of the affective disorders (Angst, 1966). This
was an emancipating step, contrary to the theories of his teacher.

In 1933, the term 'schizoaffective psychosis' was born. The father of this term is the
American psychiatrist John Kasanin, who used it in his paper 'The schizoaffective
psychoses' in the *American Journal of Psychiatry*. There, he described nine cases

of young patients in a good general condition and with a good social adaptation who suddenly developed a dramatic psychosis displaying 'schizophrenic', as well as 'affective' symptoms (Kasanin, 1933). Some of these patients had a positive family history for affective disorders. Usually a critical life event had occurred before onset, the duration of the episodes was not long, and they had a favourable outcome. It is clear that the cases described by Kasanin do not have very much in common with what we nowadays define as 'schizoaffective disorders'. Kasanin's cases actually have many more similarities to the 'bouffée délirante', to the cycloid psychoses and to the Brief Psychotic Disorder of DSM-IV and the Acute and Transient Psychotic Disorders of ICD-10.

What we actually call 'schizoaffective disorders' were described in an almost identical way by Kurt Schneider in Germany as 'cases-in-between' ('Zwischen-Fälle') (Schneider, 1950) (English translation, 1959). The current operational definitions of schizoaffective disorders in ICD-10 and DSM-IV are given in Table 2.9 and Table 2.10.

The modern definitions of schizoaffective disorders according to DSM-IV and ICD-10 are not sufficient to define all the groups and subgroups of schizoaffective disorders. These definitions are not adequate to describe and define the 'schizoaffective phenomenon'. The most important points of criticism against the definitions of DSM-IV and ICD-10 are the following. Firstly, there is no argument for the chronological distinction regarding the co-existence of schizophrenic and affective symptomatology. Secondly, neither diagnostic system involves the longitudinal aspect in their definitions. Nevertheless, one important element is common to all definitions of schizoaffective disorders: patients must fulfil the full criteria of a major depressive or manic episode and show schizophrenic symptoms.

It is now well established that schizoaffective disorders must be divided into unipolar and bipolar types, in exactly the same way as the pure affective disorders. Bipolar Schizoaffective Disorders have similar premorbid and sociodemographic features. They also have similar patterns of course and a similar response to treatment and prophylaxis as the pure affective bipolar disorders. They differ significantly from unipolar schizoaffective disorders in the same way as unipolar affective disorders differ from bipolar affective disorders (Marneros et al., 1989a,b, 1990a, b, 1991b).

From a clinical point of view, schizoaffective disorders are, in spite of some overlaps, not identical to ICD-10 ATPD or DSM-IV 'Brief Psychosis'. The mandatory presence of a full affective syndrome is the most important defining element that separates schizoaffective disorders from Brief and Acute Psychoses. But they are also not identical to 'cycloid', 'reactive', 'atypical' psychoses or 'bouffée délirante' (Leonhard, 1983; Perris, 1986; Pichot, 1986a; Strömgren, 1986; Perris and Eisemann, 1989).

Table 2.9. The definition of Schizoaffective Disorder (F25) according to ICD-10

Note. This diagnosis depends upon an approximate 'balance' between the number, severity, and duration of the schizophrenic and affective symptoms.

G1 The disorder meets the criteria for one of the affective disorders (F30, F31, F32) of moderate or severe degree, as specified for each category.

G2 Symptoms from at least one of the groups listed below must be clearly present for most of the time during a period of at least 2 weeks:

- thought echo, thought insertion or withdrawal, thought broadcasting
- delusions of control, influence, or passivity, clearly referred to body or limb movements or specific thoughts, actions, or sensations
- hallucinatory voices giving a running commentary on the patient's behaviour or discussing the patient among themselves, or other types of hallucinatory voices coming from some part of the body
- persistent delusions of other kinds that are culturally inappropriate and completely impossible, but not merely grandiose or persecutory (criterion G1(1)d for F20.0-F20.3), e.g. has visited other worlds; can control the clouds by breathing in and out; can communicate with plants or animals without speaking
- grossly irrelevant or incoherent speech, or frequent use of neologisms
- intermittent but frequent appearance of some forms of catatonic behaviour, such as posturing, waxy flexibility and negativism

G3 Criteria G1 and G2 above must be met within the same episode of the disorder, and concurrently for at least part of the episode. Symptoms from both G1 and G2 must be prominent in the clinical picture.

G4 Most commonly used exclusion clause. The disorder is not attributable to organic mental disorder (in the sense of F00–F09), or to psychoactive substance-related intoxication, dependence, or withdrawal (F10–F19).

Brief and Acute Psychoses as side products of epidemiological studies

Systematic epidemiological studies regarding Acute and Transient Psychotic Disorders or Brief Psychotic Disorder are rare and exist practically only as 'side-products' of epidemiological studies on schizophrenia or other mental disorders. The most important of these is discussed below. The *ICD-10 Field Study* (Sartorius *et al.*, 1995), designed to evaluate the ICD-10 Diagnostic Criteria for Research in 151 centres in 32 countries, found that within 1186 diagnoses of the chapter F2 (schizophrenia, schizotypal and delusional disorders), 135 patients were diagnosed as having ATPD. This amounts to 11.4%. Among these, 92 patients (i.e. 7.8%) were diagnosed with Acute Polymorphic Psychosis.

The relatively high frequency of ATPD in the WHO population (especially in comparison to the findings of the *Halle Study on Brief and Acute Psychoses*–HASBAP

Table 2.10. Diagnostic criteria for Schizoaffective Disorder (295.70) according to DSM-IV

Note. The Major Depressive Episode must include Criterion A1: depressed mood.

A. An uninterrupted period of illness during which, at some time, there is either a Major Depressive Episode, a Manic Episode, or a Mixed Episode concurrent with symptoms that meet Criterion A for Schizophrenia.

B. During the same period of illness, there have been delusions or hallucinations for at least 2 weeks in the absence of prominent mood symptoms.

C. Symptoms that meet criteria for a mood episode are present for a substantial portion of the total duration of the active and residual periods of the illness.

D. The disturbance is not due to the direct physiological effects of a substance (e. g. a drug of abuse, a medication) or a general medical condition.

Specify type

Bipolar Type: if the disturbance includes a Manic or a Mixed Episode (or a Manic or a Mixed Episode and Major Depressive Episodes)

Depressive Type: if the disturbance only includes Major Depressive Episodes

---

– see p. 72) could be explained by the inclusion of the so-called developing countries. The frequency of ATPD in developing countries seems to be significantly higher than in developed industrial European and North-American countries (Jilek and Jilek-Aall, 1970; German, 1972; Cooper and Sartorius, 1977; Stevens, 1987; Wig and Parhee, 1988; Cooper *et al.*, 1990; Verma *et al.*, 1992; Okasha *et al.*, 1993; Manton *et al.*, 1994; Susser and Wanderling, 1994; Collins *et al.*, 1996; Das *et al.*, 2001). A part of the literature on the frequency of Brief, as well as Acute and Transient Psychotic Disorder, in developing countries is based on case reports or non-representative reviews. Relevant information, however, can also be found in some systematic studies mostly initiated by the WHO (the 'International Pilot Study on Schizophrenia', IPSS, the 'Determinance of Outcome of Severe Mental Disorder Study', DOSMD, and the 'Cross-Cultural Study of Acute Psychoses').

In the *International Pilot Study on Schizophrenia* (IPSS, WHO, 1979), 1202 patients with so-called 'endogenous psychoses' were uniformly investigated. The study was carried out in nine countries (Colombia, Czechoslovakia, Denmark, India, Nigeria, China, Russia, United Kingdom, USA). One of the most important findings of this study was that the schizophrenic patients in the centres of developing countries (Nigeria, India, Colombia) had a more favourable course and 2-year outcome than patients in centres of industrial countries.

In a re-analysis of the IPSS data applying a statistical model, eight 'pure types' of diagnostic classes were identified. One of them, characterised by paranoid-hallucinatory symptoms, hyperactivity, aggression, disorganised behaviour, short duration and favourable prognosis, was found to be more frequent in patients in the developing countries (Manton *et al.*, 1994). The more favourable prognosis of schizophrenic disorders in the developing countries, found by the IPSS, could result from a variety of factors, including sociological, cultural or even symptomatological factors (Cooper and Sartorius, 1977). A possible interpretation is that the diagnostic system (PSE/CATEGO) pays no attention to the duration of the psychotic symptoms, so that the overrepresentation of Brief Psychoses in the developing countries contributed to the hyperproportionality of favourable prognosis. However, according to DSM criteria such psychoses could not be diagnosed as schizophrenia (Stevens, 1987).

The *Determinants of Outcome of Severe Mental Disorder Study* (DOSMED, Jablensky *et al.*, 1992; Susser and Wanderling, 1994) investigated the prognostic aspect. From the voluminous ICD-9 schizophrenia, a group of 'Non-affective Acute Remitting Psychosis' (NARP) was separated. The most important defining features of NARP were onset within 1 week without prodromal syndromes and complete remission. The incidence of NARP in developing countries was approximately ten times higher than in the industrial countries. Females were represented significantly more frequently than males. No difference regarding the age at onset between females and males was found. Susser and Wanderling (1994) discussed the possibility that the NARP are the benign form of schizophrenia, but they prefer a nosological independence of this group.

The *Cross-Cultural Study of Acute Psychoses* was initiated by the WHO and carried out using the Schedule for Clinical Assessment of Acute Psychotic States (SCAAPS). The investigators found a full remission after 1 year in 80% of patients with acute psychoses (broad definition), but the interpretation of these results is hampered by methodological problems and by an unequal quality of data between centres (Cooper *et al.*, 1990). In a substudy, Okasha (1993) in Cairo examined 85 acute psychotic patients applying the SCAAPS. The diagnoses were made not only according to SCAAPS (i.e. ICD-9 diagnoses), but also according DSM-III and ICD-10. 74% of patients were diagnosed as having an Acute and Transient Psychotic Disorder (ATPD). The diagnoses remained relatively stable so that after 1 year only 20% of the patients had to be rediagnosed with schizophrenia. The investigation of Verma and co-workers (1992) in Chandirgarh in India showed that 40% of patients having a psychotic disorder could not be allocated into the CATEGO categories 'schizophrenia' or 'affective disorder'. The authors advocated the creation of a category called 'Acute and Transient Psychotic Disorders'.

Findings supporting the assumption that Acute and Transient Psychotic Disorders are overrepresented in groups of immigrants from developing countries in comparison to the native population (Littlewood and Lipsedge, 1981; Johnson-

Sabine *et al.*, 1983) could not be replicated by other studies, for example by the Nottingham Study (Harrison *et al.*, 1988).

Conclusion: There is consistent evidence from epidemiological studies of an elevated frequency of Brief and Acute Psychoses in developing countries. Most of these findings, however, are 'side-products' of epidemiological studies, and need to be validated by prospective observations of patients with Brief and Acute Psychoses diagnosed according to standardised criteria.

Part II

Studies and findings

3

Studies on brief and acute psychoses

This chapter describes the few studies that have investigated samples of patients with ATPD according to ICD-10 or BP according to DSM-IV only. The characteristics of the patients' samples, the methods of the studies and the principal results are mentioned here. More detailed results and their discussions, however, are reported in the appropriate sections of Chapters 4 to 10. A particular emphasis is on the Halle Study on Brief and Acute Psychoses, the most extensive study so far. At the beginning of this chapter, we also consider a number of studies using modified criteria. These studies have addressed the problem of Acute Brief Psychoses explicitly, and they provide data that have bearing on current and future operational criteria of ATPD and BP. Most of these investigations are based on international studies conducted by the WHO, some of which have already been mentioned on page 37 ff. In accordance with the high prevalence of Acute Brief Psychoses in developing countries, much of the relevant data have been collected from there. India, in particular, is a country where a good deal of research on Acute Brief Psychoses has been done.

Studies using modified criteria of Brief and Acute Psychoses

As we have seen above, ICD-10 and DSM-IV have given different sets of diagnostic criteria for Brief and Acute Psychoses. A number of studies, some of which were designed and conducted before publication of ICD-10 and DSM-IV, have used their own operational criteria differing both from ICD-10 and DSM-IV. These 'modified' criteria deviate from the ICD-10 and DSM-IV criteria, mainly in terms of duration, and some of them also demand a certain pattern of course. The following paragraph discusses the results of the studies using such modified criteria of Brief and Acute Psychoses.

Re-analyses of the WHO DOSMED cohort

In the first of a series of papers, Susser and co-workers (1994) re-analysed data from the WHO *Determinants of Outcome of Severe Mental Disorder Study* (DOSMED)

(Jablensky *et al.*, 1992). In this study, in 13 defined catchment areas in several countries (Agra, India; Cali, Columbia; urban Chandigarh, rural Chandigarh, India; Ibadan, Nigeria; Aarhus, Denmark; Dublin, Ireland; Honolulu, Hawai; Moscow, Russia; Nagasaki, Japan; Nottingham, England; Prague, the Czech Republic; Rochester, USA) over a 2-year period, all patients aged 15–54 years with a psychotic illness were investigated at their first contact with an aide agency. It turned out that in only 8 of the 13 sites were the findings sufficiently complete to calculate incidence rates. This was the case in two developing country sites (rural Chandigarh and urban Chandigarh) and in six industrialised country sites (Aarhus, Dublin, Honolulu, Moscow, Nagasaki and Nottingham). Patients were followed up for 2 years.

In their analysis of the DOSMED data, Susser and co-workers (1994) defined the category of Non-affective Acute Remitting Psychoses (NARP) as those with (1) acute onset as defined by the development of a psychotic state within one week without any prodrome and (2) a remitting course as evidenced by single psychotic episode followed by a complete remission or two or more psychotic episodes with complete remission between all or most of the episodes. Complete remission meant 'the patient is virtually symptom free and shows his or her usual premorbid personality'.

For all centres, the sex ratio of incidence rates and the gender specific age at onset were determined. The results of this study showed that the incidence of NARP in developing countries was ten times higher than in industrialised countries. In both settings, the sex ratio was biased in favour of women. The typical gender difference in age at onset was found for non-NARP schizophrenia, but not for NARP. In the discussion, the authors considered the possibility that NARP are a benign subform of schizophrenia, but preferred nosological independence, which they saw as being supported by the lack of gender difference in age at onset.

Susser and co-workers (1998) reported 12-year follow-up data for particular subgroups of the Chandigarh sample in the WHO DOSMED study. Index diagnosis was based on the data collected at intake and at 2-year follow-up. In this study, the criteria for Non-Affective Acute Remitting Psychoses (NARP), now called 'Acute Brief Psychoses', were refined (i.e. made more strict) by the authors when compared to the earlier definition cited above (Susser and Wanderling, 1994; Susser *et al.*, 1996). In particular, early relapse (up to 2 years after onset) was no longer allowed, otherwise a diagnosis of acute relapsing psychosis was assigned. In addition, an affective episode within 2 years after the index episode was an exclusion criterion. At the 12-year follow-up, 17 of the initial 20 patients with Acute Brief Psychoses could be investigated with the Present State Examination and several WHO instruments. Their course and outcome was compared to 36 (of initially 43) patients with other forms of remitting psychoses. At that time, retrospective ICD-10 diagnoses were also assigned according to the index episode. At the 12-year follow-up, only 1 of 17 patients (6%) with Acute Brief Psychoses was still considered to be ill, in contrast to 18 of 36 patients (50%) with other remitting psychoses ($P = 0.002$ in Fisher's exact test). Psychotic relapses had occurred in the non-recovered patients in 2 of the 16 recovered patients with Acute Brief Psychoses; none of these patients had an affective episode during follow-up. Re-diagnosis of the index episode according to ICD-10 resulted in 11 cases of schizophrenia, 3 of Other Acute and Transient Psychotic Disorder, 2 with Acute Schizophrenia-like Psychotic Disorder and 1 with another non-organic psychotic disorder.

Another study (Collins *et al.*, 1996), explored biological and psychosocial contributions to the incidence of Acute Brief Psychoses in three developing country sites. The study used data from 5-year follow-up investigations in Ibadan, Nigeria and Agra, India (patients recruited in the International Pilot Study of Schizophrenia) and in rural Chandigarh (patients recruited in the DOSMED). Baseline narratives of the cases and controls were reviewed and rated for presence or absence of three exposures: fever, departure from or return to the parental village for women, and job distress for men. Results showed an association between fever and Acute Brief Psychosis in all three sites. There was an association between Acute Brief Psychosis and departure from or return to the parental village among women in all sites, and among men, an association between job distress and Acute Brief Psychosis was noted in Ibadan and Agra. The authors concluded that psychosocial and biological factors such as these three exposures merit further research to clarify their roles in the aetiology of Acute Brief Psychoses.

Collins and co-workers (1999) analysed a special subsample of the DOSMED cohort that was part of the Life Events Substudy and consisted of 67 patients from rural and urban Chandigarh with a non-affective ICD-9 diagnosis, who were followed up for 12 months. A modified definition of NARP was used, demanding no affective syndrome and freedom of relapse during 12 months, instead of 24 months, since 24-month follow-up data were not available for this subsample. Seventeen patients met this definition. They were compared with 40 patients from this cohort with acute or subacute psychoses but not fulfilling the criteria of NARP. In the NARP sample, 8 of 17 patients had antecedent fever during the 12 weeks before onset, while among the controls, 5 of 40 patients had antecedent fever, yielding an odds ratio of 6.2.

The most recent re-analysis of DOSMED data was undertaken by Mojtabai (2000). In contrast to the 1994 study (Susser and Wanderling, 1994), not only were the 8 'incidence sites' of the DOSMED, but all 13 sites were included. The analysis started with the 794 patients that had a full initial evaluation, a 2-year follow-up assessment, an ICD-9 diagnosis of schizophrenia at study entry and no clear-cut affective syndrome during the follow-up period. They defined 'remitting psychoses with acute onset' as psychotic disorders with acute onset, complete remission and no relapses within the 2-year follow-up period. Of note, in this analysis remission could occur at any point during the 24 months of follow-up. This definition allowed the authors to not only calculate gender ratio and the relative frequency of the 'remitting psychoses with acute onset' in developing vs. industrialised countries, but also to calculate the duration of the episode. The authors found that many of the 'remitting psychoses with acute onset' had a duration exceeding 3 months. They suggested that the ICD-10 criteria for ATPD be revised.

Re-analysis of the Suffolk County Mental Health Project

The study of Susser and co-workers (1995a) used data from the Suffolk County Mental Health Project in New York. In this study, a large cohort of patients with first-onset affective and non-affective psychotic disorders aged 15–60 were followed-up and investigated with the Structured Clinical Interview for DSM-III-R (SCID). Two hundred and twenty-one first-admission patients were given extensive assessments at initial evaluation, a 6-month follow-up and a 24-month follow-up. The research team made consensus ratings of the presence of psychosis, DSM-III-R diagnosis, mode of onset of disorder, and course of disorder. Brief Psychoses were defined by a diagnosis of non-affective psychosis at the initial evaluation and a rating of full remission at the 6-month follow-up; Acute Brief Psychoses met the additional criterion of acute onset as defined by ICD-10. Of the sample of 221 patients, 20 patients (9%) were considered to suffer from Brief Psychoses. Only 7 patients (3%) were diagnosed with Acute Brief Psychoses. Among these, six occurred in women, and none had evolved into an affective disorder or a chronic disorder by the time of the 24-month follow-up. The 13 non-Acute Brief Psychoses had a more equal gender distribution (7/13 female). Two of these had one episode with full remission, six had multiple episodes with full remissions and five had multiple episodes without full remissions. Two were rediagnosed as having affective disorders at the 24-month follow-up. The authors concluded that Acute Brief Psychoses emerged as a highly distinctive and temporally stable form of psychosis that may merit a separate diagnostic classification. They also conjectured that the more numerous non-Acute Brief Psychoses may represent mild forms of non-affective psychoses such as schizophrenia.

Conclusions and consequences

The above-mentioned studies on 'Non-Affective Remitting Psychoses' in their varying definitions have yielded remarkable results, but they also suffer from important limitations. One of the most striking findings of the trans-national studies was the verification of the long-suspected intercultural variations in incidence. These variations may lead to an up to ten-fold higher incidence of acute and brief psychoses in developing countries as compared with industrialised countries. The reasons for this difference still remain essentially obscure, but they are of high theoretical and practical importance. Another important finding was that several studies have highlighted the importance of the criterion of 'acute onset' as an obligatory feature for Brief and Acute Psychoses (Susser *et al.*, 1995a, 1996). An important limitation of all studies reported so far derives from the fact that the diagnostic criteria employed differ from the internationally accepted classification systems ICD-10 and DSM-IV, and also differ between the individual studies. In particular, the criterion requiring absence of any relapse within 2 years after the index episode was somewhat arbitrary. It was in part motivated by the fact that the DOSMED study did not contain data on the duration of relapses occurring during the 2-year follow-up period, i.e. the occurrence of another Acute Brief Psychosis during this time could not be distinguished from the occurrence of longer psychotic episodes (Mojtabai *et al.*, 2000). However, most researchers would still assign a diagnosis of Acute Brief Psychosis if a patient, after full remission, has another episode of an Acute Brief Psychosis one and a half years after the index episode. In the study of Collins and co-workers (1999), only 1 year without relapse was required because only 1-year follow-up data were available. These discrepancies highlight the difficulties associated with diagnostic criteria requiring freedom of relapse during a specified period of time: the arbitrariness of the criteria and the practical difficulty that diagnosis is impossible in patients without sufficient follow-up data. The point made by Mojtabai, Susser and colleagues (Mojtabai *et al.*, 2000) that many Acute Brief Psychoses may have more than one, and even more than 2 months' duration is well worth considering. At the present state, however, it would be very problematic to define Acute Brief Psychoses in a way that leads to overlap with ICD-10 or DSM-IV schizophrenia. In this case, a substantial number of patients up to now diagnosed with schizophrenia in ICD and DSM would have to be re-classified, and a comparison with earlier studies no longer would be possible. To avoid this, ICD-10 and DSM-IV have set the time criteria for ATPD and BP in a way that prevents an overlap with schizophrenia. We now turn to studies using these definitions.

Studies on ICD-10 ATPD

The Cairo study

Okasha and co-workers (1993) in Cairo conducted a study on acute psychotic disorders using the Schedule of Clinical Assessment of Acute Psychotic States (SCAAPS) as developed by the WHO (Cooper *et al.*, 1990). Patients were recruited from 1987 to 1989 from two Cairo hospitals, and inclusion criteria were rather wide: the start of psychotic or major affective symptoms within 3 months before initial assessment, preceded by a state of apparent mental health for at least 3 months. The SCAAPS included symptom checklists and sections dealing with psychiatric history, treatment, course and outcome. The patients were followed up for 1 year, but only 50 of 85 patients were still in the study after 1 year. Seventy-four per cent of the final sample were reported as ATPD on initial contact, 54% had this diagnosis after 1 year, but 20% of the patients had to be rediagnosed with schizophrenia. Sixty-four per cent of the whole sample were symptom-free at the 1-year follow-up assessment. Although the methodology of this study has important limitations, in connection with other findings it substantiated the necessity to include a category for Acute and Transient Psychotic Disorders in ICD-10.

The cohort study of Chandigarh, India

Das and co-workers (1999) conducted a family study on 40 probands with ATDP and 40 patients with ICD-10 schizophrenia at the Psychiatric Department of the Post Graduate Institute of Medical Education and Research in Chandigarh, India. They recruited the probands between 1994 and 1995 on the basis of ICD-10 criteria, although they did not use a structured interview. The availability for interview of at least three first-degree relatives (FDR) was a necessary precondition for inclusion. FDRs were interviewed using a modified version of the Family History Assessment module, a semi-structured interview schedule originally developed in St Louis for the Collaborative Study on the Genetics of Alcoholism. The modified version of the instrument included questions to elicit ICD-10 research diagnoses including ATPD and schizotypical personality disorder. Age, sex, socio-economic status, locality (urban/rural), marital status, religion, family type (nuclear/joint), clinical diagnosis and duration of illness were recorded for all patients. FDR between 15 and 45 years of age were interviewed personally by the first author, who was not blind to the proband diagnoses.

The main result of this study was that FDRs of ATP probands had a higher prevalence of ATPD than those of schizophrenic probands. FDRs of schizophrenic probands had significantly higher prevalence of schizophrenia than those of ATP probands. ATPD subtypes with schizophrenic symptomatology (ICD-10 codes F 23.1 and F 23.2) had more family history of schizophrenia than the rest of the ATP subtypes. The authors concluded that ATPD had a differential pattern of risk of illness compared to schizophrenia and that the subtypes subsumed under ICD-10 ATPD may be genetically heterogeneous.

In a companion publication, Das and co-workers (2001) reported a negative association between stressful life events and a family history of psychiatric disorders in the ATPD sample. Stressful life events during the year preceding the onset of ATPD were recorded with the 'Presumptive Stressful Life Events Scale' (PSLES), a 51-item scale with accompanying stress scores for each event, developed for use in the north Indian population. Thirteen of the 40 ATPD probands were considered family-history positive (in contrast to the analysis reported above, four relatives with an 'unspecified' disorder were included, one proband had two affected relatives), 27 were family-history negative. Stressful life events within 2 weeks prior to the onset of ATPD were experienced by 11 of the FHN probands and by 2 of the FHP probands (no significant difference). When life events within 1 year before the onset of ATPD were considered, there was a significant difference both in the total number of life events and in the total stress score. The authors interpret this result as supporting the vulnerability stress hypothesis in the aetiology of ATPD.

The cohort study of Pondicherry, India

Sajith and co-workers (2002) recruited consecutive patients from the Department of Psychiatry at JIPMER Hospital, Pondicherry, India, meeting ICD-10 research criteria for ATPD, polymorphic subtype without symptoms of schizophrenia (F23.0). All patients were recruited between April 1997 and March 1998. In addition to meeting ICD-10 research criteria for Acute Polymorphic Psychotic Disorder, patients had to be 15–60 years old and experiencing their first episode of a psychotic illness. Patients with evidence of an organic aetiology including epilepsy, with evidence of current alcohol/substance dependence or withdrawal and with a duration of the illness of more than 1 month at the time of first contact with the hospital were excluded. Assessment was done using the following instruments: (1) a semistructured proforma to record demographic details, family data and course of the illness; (2) the Comprehensive Psychopathological Rating Scale; (3) presence and severity of a preceding psychosocial stressor according to axis IV of DSM-III-R and stress during the 2 weeks prior to the onset of psychosis according to the criteria for ATPD in ICD-10; (4) the Global Assessment of Functioning (GAF) Scale. The criterion of full remission within 3 months was operationalised by the authors as achieving at least 80% of the premorbid GAF score. Fifty-two of 58 patients initially considered for inclusion met this criterion. Patients were reassessed at 1 month, 3 months, 6 months and at the end of 3 years. Revision of diagnosis was attempted at each stage of assessment using the ICD-10 criteria. Three-year follow-up data were available for 45 of the 52 patients.

The main results of the study were as follows: There was a marked female preponderance in the sample with 71.1% female patients. The mean age was 26.9 years without any significant gender difference. Onset was abrupt (within 48 h) for 30 patients (66.7%) and acute (>48 h but <2 weeks) for 15 patients (33.3%). Fifteen patients (33.3%) had a family history of psychotic illness in their first-degree relatives, but information was inadequate to determine the exact diagnoses of secondary cases. The duration of the index episode was less than 1 month in 24 (53.3%) patients and between 1 and 3 months in 21 (46.7%) patients. Auditory hallucinations and delusions of persecution were seen in most patients (91.1% and

82.2%, respectively), although schizophrenic first-rank symptoms were excluded in this sample by definition. Stress within 2 weeks prior to the onset of psychosis was present in 31 (68.9%) patients. At the end of 3 years, 33 (73.3%) patients retained their index diagnosis of Acute Polymorphic Psychotic Disorder, 24 of these had no further episode. Ten patients (22.2%) were re-diagnosed as having bipolar affective disorder, and two patients (4.4%) had a diagnostic revision to unspecified non-organic psychosis. A shorter duration of the index episode (<1 months and an abrupt onset (<48 h) predicted a stable diagnosis of ATPD. None of the other base-line characteristics, including gender, age, presence of preceding stress or symptoms at first contact, showed statistically significant association with diagnostic stability. Patients retaining a diagnosis of Acute Polymorphic Psychotic Disorder had a significantly better outcome in terms of the Global Assessment of Functioning Score. The authors view their results as favouring a separate diagnostic entity of Acute Polymorphic Psychotic Disorder.

The Danish retrospective study

From 1984–1992 Pavl Jørgensen in Denmark conducted a large longitudinal study on first admitters with delusional beliefs and no organic disorder (Jørgensen and Jensen 1994a,b,c, Jørgensen 1994a,b). ICD-10 diagnoses were made retrospectively and included a subgroup with ATPD. Among 548 first admissions of the year 1984 in Aarhus/Risskov, 88 patients with delusional symptoms were identified. Patients with an organic disorder were excluded. The patients were interviewed at the index admission, in 1986, in 1988 and in 1992. Initial assessment included the present state examination, PSE-9, and the main delusional theme (persecution, reference, influence including primary delusions, guilt, other delusions). In 1988, the Global Assessment of Functioning (DSM) was determined, as well as the delusional beliefs in a dimensional way. In 1992, diagnoses according to DSM-III-R and ICD-10 were made by use of the Schedules for Clinical Assessment in Neuropsychiatry (SCAN). Social outcome was assessed with the McGlashan scale. Of the 88 patients, 17 were judged to have ATPD (other diagnoses: 43 schizophrenia, 19 affective disorders, 9 delusional disorder). With regard to ATPD, the following findings emerged: the main delusional theme were delusions of reference (10/17 patients), while in schizophrenia, persecution and influence were predominant (23 and 13 of 43 patients, respectively) (Jørgensen and Jensen, 1994a). Among the patients who were available for follow-up investigations ($n = 75$), those with ATPD had a favourable outcome according to GAF (mean score 72) when compared to schizophrenia (mean score 35), affective disorders (mean score 82) and persistent delusional disorder (mean score 50). Similar differences were found with the Disability Assessment Schedule and with the global-course scores according to McGlashan. Diagnostic change occurred in only a few cases. Of the whole group, only eight patients changed diagnosis from the index episode to the 8-year follow-up (Jørgensen, 1994b). Of the ATPD patients, 87% remained diagnostically stable (Jørgensen, 1995). Limitations of the study are the retrospective design and incomplete characterisation of the diagnostic groups, e.g. with regard to socio-demographic data.

The Danish cohort study

Jørgensen and co-workers (1996) recruited a sample of 51 inpatients at the Psychiatric Hospital in Aarhus (Department A, Psychiatric Hospital, Risskov, Denmark) who fulfilled the ICD-10 research diagnostic criteria for ATPD during the period between May 1994 and June 1995. Patients who previously fulfilled the diagnostic criteria for organic mental disorder, mental disorder due to psychoactive substance use, schizophrenia or affective disorder, were excluded. Within the first 1–2 weeks of admission, the patients' mental state was assessed with the OPCRIT system (McGuffin et al., 1991), which includes a criteria checklist for psychotic disorders and a computer program for the generation of DSM diagnoses. Patients were monitored during their admission and re-interviewed when they were in a non-psychotic state. The authors assessed (1) social and vocational activity during the year before admission according to the McGlashan scale; (2) the Global assessment of functioning during the previous year; (3) the presence and severity of a preceding psychosocial stressor according to DSM-III-R axis IV; (4) the International Personality Disorder Examination to assess the presence of DSM-IV and ICD-10 personality disorders.

The main results of the study of Jørgensen and co-workers (1996) can be summarised as follows. There was a marked female preponderance with a female/male ratio of 3.3. The mean age at the index episode was 37 years, with males being on average somewhat younger than females (mean age at index episode for female patients was 39 years, for male patients 30 years). The mean age at onset was 33 years (range 18–65 years). Two-thirds of the patients belonged to the polymorphic subtypes of ATPD. Associated stress within 2 weeks before onset was present in 53% of patients, but a severe stressor was only found in 3 patients (11% of patients with life events). Concordance with DSM-IV diagnoses was calculated with Schizophreniform Disorder, Brief Psychotic Disorder and Psychotic Disorder Not Otherwise Specified being applicable in descending frequency. Only 10% of the patients did not receive medication at initial assessment. The International Personality Disorder Examination revealed a high prevalence (63%) of comorbid personality disorders. However, ATPD was not related to any specific personality disorders; unspecified personality disorder was by far the most frequent personality disorder in the patients investigated.

One year after the index episode, follow-up investigations were conducted using personal interviews ($n = 43$) or telephone interviews ($n = 3$). A diagnostic classification was performed using ICD-10 and DSM-IV criteria. In addition, the presence of a personality disorder and several aspects of psychosocial functioning (hospitalisation, social contacts, work, psychopathology, global functioning) were assessed. Of the five dropouts, two had emigrated, two did not want to participate, one had died of causes not associated with the mental disorder. During the 1-year period of follow-up, 15 patients (33%) had been re-admitted because of a psychotic relapse. Non-psychotic relapses and non-re-admitted relapses were not assessed. Three of the 15 patients had another ATPD. The authors concluded that, when all of the available information was taken into consideration, the diagnostic category was changed for 22 patients (48%) and unchanged for 24 patients (52%). Diagnostic change was most often to schizophrenia (15%) and to affective disorder (28%). When personality disorders were re-assessed they were found to be considerably less frequent than at the first follow-up. When baseline characteristics were compared between patients still believed to be ATPD at follow-up ($n = 24$) and those who where not ($n = 22$), no significant differences were found with regard to gender, age, occupational and social adjustment, GAF, psychosocial stressors, presence of a personality disorder, abrupt onset, polymorphic clinical picture or a diagnosis of DSM-IV Brief Psychosis.

From index admission to follow-up, patients with an unchanged diagnosis of ATPD managed fairly well with regard to psychosocial functioning, and no deteriorating development was observed. The authors stress the need for validation of the concept of ATPD, and point to the fact that brief psychotic episodes with an acute onset may be an early manifestation of severe mental disorder (schizophrenia and affective disorder).

Other studies on ATPD

In the course of ICD-10 field studies, inter-rater reliability studies were performed. Albus and co-workers (Albus *et al.*, 1990), in the German field trial of the ICD-10 draft, found an inter-rater reliability for the diagnosis of ATPD of 0.82. Reliability values of the international study, however, yielded less favourable values (Sartorius *et al.*, 1995).

Some case reports on ATPD have been published. Schär and co-workers (1995) conducted SPECT investigations in psychotic patients including three subjects with ATPD and did not find any differences between ATPD and schizophrenia in a measure of hypofrontality. Murai and co-workers (1996) reported a patient with ATPD who was repeatedly assessed using a brief neuropsychological assessment during his recovery from the psychotic episode. Characteristic findings, including impairment of attention tests, dysgraphia and constructional disturbances, were seen during the psychotic period, but improved with recovery on a behavioural level. The authors discussed the similarity of neuropsychological and behavioural abnormalities of this patient and those of patients in an acute confusional state. Strömgren reported on a series of patients, including two with ATPD, who have been successfully treated with ACT in Aarhus psychiatric hospital (Strömgren 1997). In Sao Paulo, Brazil, Pitta and Blay (1997) conducted a case note study to evaluate the agreement between the diagnoses of reactive and hysterical psychosis obtained using ICD-9 criteria with those obtained using the DSM-III-R, DSM-IV, ICD-10 and PSE diagnostic systems. The main result of the study was that the operationalised criteria sets, including ATPD, did not show a good concordance with the concept of psychogenic (reactive) psychoses. Iwawaki and co-workers (1996) in Japan described two cases of ATPD (polymorphic subtype in adults with mild intellectual deficits). They discussed pathogenetic aspects and concluded that, with their low self-esteem, precipitating events forced the patients to act inappropriately and, as a result, they became psychotic. The cohort study of Amin and co-workers (Amin *et al.*, 1999) on diagnostic stability in first-episode psychosis included 30 patients with ICD-10 ATPD. After 3 years, 11 of these patients were still assigned a diagnosis of ATPD.

Studies on BP

Systematic studies on Brief Psychotic Disorders are virtually absent from the psychiatric literature with the exception of a few case reports. Abe and co-workers (Abe *et al.*, 1998) reported on a case of hypogammaglobulinemia in a 22-year-old woman treated with antipsychotics for brief psychotic disorder. Chiniwala and co-workers (Chiniwala *et al.*, 1996) described a patient with Brief Psychotic Disorder presenting as 'Koro'. To date, no systematic investigations on DSM-IV diagnosed Brief Psychotic Disorder have been published.

A study from Bangalor, India (Janakiramaiah *et al.*, 1998) reported on 22 male patients with DSM-IV Brief Psychotic Disorder who had blood and liquor essays for viral antibodies (cytoalomegalovirus, herpes simplex type I, mumps, measles, varicella zoster and Japanese encephalitis). Their clinical status was weekly assessed with the Brief Psychiatric Rating Scale and with the Positive and Negative Syndrome Scale. Eleven patients had viral infection as evidenced by a four-fold change in antibody titre. The duration of illness in these patients was significantly shorter than in patients without infection, usually less than 2 weeks.

Tsoh and co-workers (2000) in Singapore reported two Chinese patients who, following a brief, acute psychosis met the DSM-IV criteria of Brief Psychotic Disorder. Therapy comprised drug treatment with low dose antipsychotics and benzodiazepines, coupled with hypnosis and marital therapy to explore and treat the underlying pathology. Both psychotic states resolved. Follow-up at 12 months revealed stable mental condition in one subject; however, the second patient was lost to follow-up.

Mechri and co-workers reported 16 cases of psychotic episodes following marriage, predominantly affecting male patients (75%) (Mechri *et al.*, 2000). Episodes were mainly Schizophreniform Psychoses of Brief Psychotic Disorders. The cases were discussed in their connection to the Maghrebin cultural context particular to the study subjects.

Finally, one large longitudinal study on a first-admission sample with psychosis ($n = 547$) includes data on DSM-IV Brief Psychotic Disorder: the Suffolk County Mental Health Project (NY, USA) that has already been mentioned above (Schwartz *et al.*, 2000). The study evaluated the stability of research diagnoses by reassessment of the patients 6 and 24 months after enrolment. For diagnosis, the Structured Clinical Interview for DSM-IV was used in connection with the analysis of hospital files and data from sources. Consensus diagnoses were formulated by psychiatrists blind to previous research diagnoses. The most temporally consistent 6-month categories proved to be schizophrenia (92%), bipolar disorder (83%) and major depression (74%); the least stable were psychosis not otherwise specified (44%), schizoaffective disorder (36%) and Brief Psychosis (27%). However, the number of Brief Psychoses was very small (11 of 547 at 6 months, 6 of 547 at 24 months). The type of diagnostic change from Brief Psychosis was very variable, with only one patient being diagnosed with schizophrenia at 24 months, and another patient with Schizophreniform Disorder.

The Halle Study on Brief and Acute Psychoses (HASBAP)

The *Halle Study on Brief and Acute Psychoses* (HASBAP) is the most systematic investigation of the topic. That is why we describe it somewhat extensively. It was initiated and designed by the senior author (Andreas Marneros) and co-ordinated and managed by the second author (Frank Pillmann). As already pointed out, neither the Brief Psychosis of DSM-IV nor Acute and Transient Psychotic Disorders of ICD-10 are based on a broad ground of research. The delineation of Brief and Acute Psychoses from other psychotic disorders, especially schizophrenia or schizoaffective disorders, is of essential relevance for research and clinical work, but also for the social management and rehabilitation of patients. Therefore, the aim of the HASBAP was to answer the following questions:

1. What are the clinical, paraclinical, sociobiographical, therapeutic and prognostic features of Brief and Acute Psychoses?
2. Can their modern definition, classification, subtyping and defining criteria be supported by operational research, or do they need to be modified?
3. What are the Brief Psychotic Disorders of DSM-IV and the Acute and Transient Psychotic Disorders of ICD-10?

4. Are they independent entities? What is their relationship to other psychotic disorders, especially to schizophrenia?

The HASBAP combines three methodological approaches:

(a) the prospective approach, studying a consecutively recruited inpatient sample with a diagnosis of 'Acute and Transient Psychotic Disorder' or 'Brief Psychotic Disorder';

(b) a case control design in which every patient of the original index cohort was matched for age and gender with two clinical and one non-clinical control groups;

(c) the longitudinal approach for all three clinical groups.

The control groups comprised (a) patients with an acute episode of 'Positive' Schizophrenia, (b) patients with an acute episode of Bipolar Schizoaffective Disorder, and (c) surgical patients without any mental disorder.

While the basic aim of the HASBAP was to examine a sample of 'Brief Psychotic Disorders' ('BP') and 'Acute and Transient Psychotic Disorders' ('ATPD') that is as representative as possible, it still has the restrictions of a non-epidemiological study. It was intended to explore a large array of parameters in order to describe biographical, clinical and prognostic long-term features of ATPD, as well as to gain information relevant to their nosological status within the spectrum of non-organic psychotic and non-organic affective disorders. This objective directed the choice of control groups and the decision to match the control groups for age and gender with the index patients. Patients with schizophrenia and with Bipolar Schizoaffective Disorder were selected because the question of delineation of these disorders from ATPD and BP is of the highest relevance for conceptual reasons. The exact definition of these control groups are justified further below.

The decision to match index patients and controls for age and gender was guided by our intention to investigate possible differences between ATPD, BP and the control groups. Many features of psychotic and affective disorders are known to be mediated by age and gender. If ATPD and control groups differed in age and gender, the effects of these parameters could lead to spurious group differences in various clinical features. In this case, the differences found might not reflect true particularities of ATPD. Instead, it could be argued that any difference found would simply reflect the specific age and gender composition of the group. Such an objection could certainly be ruled out by statistical procedures, but due to the necessarily small sample size of the index group, statistical corrections might meet with difficulties. Since ATPD are rare disorders and a limited sample size had to be expected, a case control design was determined to be a more adequate way to rule out the confounding effects of age and gender.

The HASBAP includes both a 'look back' and a 'follow-up' perspective. Patients were included if they had experienced an episode of illness during the recruitment

Table 3.1. Instruments used for assessment and evaluation

- Sociobiographical interview (SBI)
- ICD-10 and DSM-IV checklists
- Schedules for Clinical Assessment in Neuropsychiatry (SCAN)
- WHO Psychological Impairments Rating Schedule (WHO/PIRS)
- WHO Disability Assessment Schedule (WHO/DAS)
- Global Assessment Scale (GAS)
- Positive and Negative Syndrome Scale (PANSS)
- NEO Five-Factor Inventory (NEO-FFI)

period and were treated for this episode at Halle University Hospital. This episode was called the index episode. The index episode was not required to be the first episode of non-organic psychotic or non-organic affective disorder in the patients. Earlier episodes were studied retrospectively, as well as sociobiographical features and family history.

A major focus of the HASBAP was the prospective investigation of the further course of the disorder beyond the index episode. Follow-up examinations were therefore performed at two time points: approximately 2 years after the index episode and approximately 5 years after the index episode. To monitor course and outcome, a broad array of standardised instruments was used, including standard scales from the large WHO studies on the course and outcome of schizophrenia (WHO, 1979; Jablensky *et al.*, 1992).

The instruments of investigation applied during the various stages of the HAS-BAP are shown in Table 3.1.

The methods and instruments of the HASBAP

The index group: Acute and Transient Psychotic Disorder and Brief Psychoses

The sample described in the HASBAP was composed of all inpatients with ATPD treated as inpatients at the Department of Psychiatry and Psychotherapy of Martin Luther University, Halle-Wittenberg from 1993 to 1997. The hospital is situated in the city of Halle, Germany and takes patients from the city as well as from the surrounding communities, which comprise both rural and industrial areas. It can be said that Halle University Hospital serves a large municipal and suburban area with a non-selective admission policy. Moreover, ATPD are acute and usually dramatic psychotic states that – considering the German health care system – nearly always lead to inpatient treatment. The sample of the HASBAP can be regarded as representative of a clinical inpatient population with ATPD. With some restrictions, the findings of this study might also be regarded – because of the above-mentioned reasons – as a reasonable approximation of ATPD in general, and not only for inpatients.

Diagnosis of ATPD according to ICD-10 or of BP according to DSM-IV can only be made after remission of the acute episode. Because of this, index diagnoses were ascertained in a two-stage fashion. Patients with a clinical discharge diagnosis of ATPD were considered for inclusion in the study. During the whole inclusion period, the hospital was directed by the senior author (A.M.). Diagnostic assessment, documentation and treatment, oriented to ICD-10, were uniform during this time. Discharge diagnoses were made by senior psychiatrists from the department under the supervision of the senior author. All patients included in the HASBAP fulfilled ICD-10 research criteria.

DSM-IV diagnoses of the index episodes were also assigned on the basis of DSM-IV criteria checklists using all available information.

The control group 'Positive Schizophrenia'

For recruitment of the psychiatric control groups, a database was used containing discharge diagnoses and demographic data on all inpatients treated at Halle University Hospital during the recruitment period. For every index patient with ATPD, a control with identical gender and a discharge diagnosis of schizophrenia was selected. The patient nearest in age to the index patient was chosen. The patient was included if the diagnosis could be confirmed by two experienced research psychiatrists applying ICD-10 checklists. To ensure comparability, only patients with an episode of 'positive' schizophrenia were selected for the schizophrenic control group. 'Positive' schizophrenia (PS) was defined as an acute episode of schizophrenia with positive symptoms, such as hallucinations or delusions. Patients with chronic schizophrenia or residual schizophrenia were excluded. The selection of patients with 'positive' schizophrenia seemed to us to be methodologically necessary because all patients with ATPD must have, by definition, positive symptoms like delusions and hallucinations. Therefore, comparisons can be made between schizophrenia and ATPD, allowing for the answer of the question: 'What are the similarities and differences between ATPD and schizophrenia'?

The control group 'Bipolar Schizoaffective Disorder'

A control group of patients with Bipolar Schizoaffective Disorder was also recruited. Only bipolar forms of schizoaffective disorder (BSAD) were included, for two reasons: Firstly, the restriction was necessary to obtain a more homogeneous sample because of the heterogeneity of schizoaffective disorder, and secondly, a bipolar characteristic of symptoms has been suggested to be an important feature in concepts of brief remitting psychoses related to ATPD. A relationship of Acute and

Transient Psychotic Disorders to bipolar disorders could be suspected from the rapid mood swings associated with the historical concepts of cycloid psychoses and bouffée délirante. More recently, experiences from the treatment response of rapid cycling mood disorders have led some authors to postulate a continuum of cycling mood disorders. This continuum is thought to range from recurrent depression to rapid cycling bipolar disorder. It is also thought to embrace recurrent catatonia and cycloid psychosis (Novac, 1998; Marneros, 1999). Within the spectrum of bipolar disorders, schizoaffective bipolar disorder would arguably be most closely related to Acute and Transient Psychotic Disorder. For a further examination of this relationship, bipolar schizoaffective patients were chosen as controls. In order to select this control group, the same procedure was used as detailed for the controls with Positive Schizophrenia.

The control group 'Mentally Healthy'

In addition, a control group of mentally healthy people was investigated. This was done to have reference data for biographical and sociopsychological features, as well as for family history data. A demographically sampled representative control group would have been preferable for this purpose. It was known, however, from previous research of the group that the acquisition of a demographically representative control group for psychiatric evaluation is very complicated within the restriction of national laws protecting privacy. Even with optimal procedures, considerable bias due to non-co-operation has to be expected. Therefore, a control group of mentally healthy subjects was recruited from inpatients of a surgical ward. Eligible subjects suffered from acute surgical illness (such as trauma, fractures, appendicitis) unrelated to any chronic medical or psychiatric condition. Patients with a history of major mental disorder or organic brain syndrome were excluded. Surgical control groups have successfully been used by earlier studies (cf. Tsuang *et al.*, 1980). Surgical controls of the HASBAP were matched for age and gender with the index patients. In rating functional status, the time period preceding the acute surgical illness was considered.

Assessment of the index episode

All data regarding the pre-episodic period, as well as the episode period and the discharge status, were recorded during the treatment period of the patients and completed if it was necessary during the follow-up, as well as through information obtained from the patient's relatives.

These features included the day of the first appearance (called the beginning of the psychotic period) of definite psychotic symptoms (e.g. hallucinations, delusions, severe derailment of thought), as well as the date when psychotic symptoms definitively disappeared (called the end of the psychotic period). The time in between was called the duration of the psychotic period.

Associated *acute stress* was rated as present according to ICD-10 criteria in a restrictive fashion (i.e. only when the first psychotic symptoms had occurred within 2 weeks of one or more events that would be regarded as stressful to most people in similar circumstances). The *acuity* of the index episode was rated as specified in the ICD-10 definition of ATPD. According to this definition, the mode of onset was determined with regard to the time period from a clearly non-psychotic state to a definitely psychotic state. Unspecific prodromal symptoms were not included, but were recorded separately.

For the evaluation of psychopathological parameters during the index episode, a symptom list was used derived from the present state examination (PSE, Wing *et al.*, 1974) and the AMDP system (AMDP, 1995). These items have been supplemented by items of specific interest in ATPD:

- 'ecstatic mood',
- 'preoccupation with religious topics',
- 'dream-like experiences',
- 'overwhelming anxiety',
- 'preoccupation with death',
- 'rapidly changing delusional topics',
- 'rapidly changing mood',
- 'rapidly changing other symptoms', and
- 'bipolarity of symptoms during episode'.

The complete list comprised 178 psychopathological items. For purposes of analysis, a number of items were aggregated into comprehensive categories: all psychotic symptoms, affective disturbance, delusions, disturbance of drive and psychomotor disturbances, thought disorder, hallucinations, euphoria, anxiety, depressed mood, and first-rank symptoms of schizophrenia.

Assessment of sociobiographical data

Sociobiographical features were evaluated using a semistructured interview already used in earlier studies (Marneros *et al.*, 1991b, 2002b; Brieger *et al.*, 2001). The interview included sections on the following topics:

- sociodemographic aspects of the primary family,
- circumstances of birth and early development,
- disruptions of the continuity of caregiving during childhood and adolescence,
- traumatic experiences,
- schooling and education,
- occupational history,
- marriage, partnership and sexual history,

- parenthood,
- living situation and social activities.

Where feasible, sociobiographical data were double-checked against information contained in the hospital files, as well as information obtained from relatives and other relevant individuals.

Family history

The HASBAP also obtained a detailed family history in order to investigate the hereditary component of ATPD. However, the relatives themselves were not investigated because after the reunification of Germany, a significant number of the East German population moved to Western Germany or abroad. Halle is located in Eastern Germany and has lost nearly 70 000 residents (at the time of reunification, 315 000 people lived in Halle and at the time of investigation, only 247 000 remained). The danger of bias (through investigating mainly 'non-mobile' relatives) was too high. Subjects were questioned about psychiatric illness in all first-degree relatives. In most cases, it was possible to make a provisional diagnosis and to differentiate between non-organic psychotic or major affective disorders and other psychiatric disorders, such as alcohol dependency, using ICD-10 criteria as a guideline. This procedure resulted, most probably, in an underestimation of the frequency of disorders. This underestimation, however, might be least pronounced for psychotic disorders, which are usually conspicuous.

Prospective follow-up

With the support of local authorities, the new addresses of patients who had moved after discharge could be located, as well as the cause and circumstances of death of those patients who had died. All living patients were contacted.

All patients were investigated and interviewed by the members of the research team (four psychiatrists and a clinical psychologist). As extensive data on illness and treatment history were obtained during the interview, investigators could not be blind to diagnosis.

Follow-up examinations of all living and consenting patients were performed. A first follow-up investigation was conducted at a mean of 8.2 years after the first episode, or 2.2 years after the index episode. Taken together, 89.7% of the original sample, or 93.4% of all surviving patients, participated in the first follow-up investigation. The investigation of the control group without mental disorders was also performed at this time.

Aiming to follow the evolution of the disorder, second follow-up examinations were performed. These second and so far last follow-up examinations took place at a mean of 4.8 (ATPD), 5.0 (PS) and 5.2 (BSAD) years after the index episode. No significant differences existed regarding the time of follow-up. This corresponds

Table 3.2. Observation time in patients with completed follow-up

	ATPD $n = 38$	PS $n = 34$	BSAD $n = 34$	
	Mean ± SD	Mean ± SD	Mean ± SD	Statistical analysis[a]
Age at follow-up	44.6 ± 11.4	44.8 ± 11.0	46.1 ± 10.5	n.s.
Time from first episode to 2nd follow-up in years	10.2 ± 7.6	10.8 ± 7.1	17.8 ± 9.7	$P < 0.001$ BSAD > ATPD** BSAD > PS**
Time from index episode to 2nd follow-up in years	4.8 ± 1.4	5.0 ± 1.3	5.2 ± 1.4	n.s.

[a] P for ANOVA, only *post-hoc* comparisons significant in Scheffé procedure are indicated.
** $P < 0.01$.
n.s. no significance.

Table 3.3. Completeness of follow-up

	ATPD	PS	BSAD
	$n(\%)$	$n(\%)$	$n(\%)$
Completed follow-up	38 (90.5)[b]	34 (80.1)[a]	34 (80.1)
Deceased	2 (4.8)	4 (9.5)	4 (9.5)
Suicide		2 (4.8)	3 (7.1)
Death from other cause	2 (4.8)	2 (4.8)	1 (2.4)
Refusal	2 (4.8)	4 (9.5)	2 (4.8)
Other reasons			2 (4.8)[c]

[a] One subject only interview with legal guardian.
[b] One subject agreed only to telephone interview.
[c] No exploration possible due to debilitating brain disease (intracerebral hemorrhage, apallic syndrome).

to a mean time of 10.2 (ATPD), 10.8 (PS) and 17.8 (BSAD) years after the first episode (details are given in Table 3.2). The healthy control group was not examined during the second follow-up because there was no reason to do it again. Table 3.3 summarises the number of subjects investigated during the last follow-up, and the reasons why the remaining subjects could not be investigated. Taken together, 84.1% of the original sample, or 91.4% of all surviving patients, participated in the last follow-up investigation. At the time of the final follow-up, two of the ATPD patients had died in the interval from natural causes, two patients refused participation and one patient consented only to detailed questioning by telephone.

The remaining 37 patients were interviewed personally. In the control group with PS, two patients had died from natural causes, and two patients had committed suicide. Four patients refused consent, and for one patient, only an information source (legal guardian) was available. The remaining 33 patients were interviewed personally. In the control group of patients with BSAD, one patient had died from a natural cause, three patients had committed suicide in the interval, two patients were unable to communicate because of severe brain damage, and two patients refused consent. The remaining 34 patients were personally interviewed. In BSAD, the patients' ages at the time of the first episode were lower than for ATPD and PS patients. BSAD patients, therefore, had a significantly longer duration of follow-up.

Characteristics of the drop-outs

Patients who dropped out did not differ significantly from patients with completed follow-up on a wide range of sociodemographic and clinical variables (diagnosis, age at first episode, educational level, family history, heterosexual partnership before onset, number of episodes, acuteness of episode, duration of episode). Patients without follow-up were significantly older at the time of the index episode (49.3 years, vs. 40.1 years, $t = 3.201$, df $= 124$, $P = 0.002$). However, this difference was only caused by the patients who had died from natural causes. When these patients were excluded from the analysis, the difference disappeared completely.

Assessment of relapses

The definition of a relapse included every remanifestation episode of non-organic psychotic and non-organic affective episodes. For the pre-recruitment period, all available information including patients' reports and case records of earlier in- and outpatient treatments at various medical care institutions were used. The case records from other hospitals or physicians were obtained with the subject's signed consent.

The use of case records was important, especially for the assessment of past episodes, because often patients' recall of dates and psychotic symptoms was poor. For past episodes, an episode definition was applied that included a treatment criterion as given below. During the follow-up period, episodes were additionally assessed episodes with a standardised interview (SCAN). Episodes assessed with SCAN were included in the analysis, independent of whether they were treated or not.

Definition of treated episodes

Past episodes of illness with in- or outpatient treatment were recorded. Any occurrence of a major affective syndrome or of psychotic symptoms severe enough either to lead to hospitalisation or to outpatient treatment was counted as an episode. To enhance reliability, outpatient episodes had to reach a certain threshold of severity as evidenced by three conditions:

- specialist treatment must have been sought,
- psychiatric medication in therapeutic doses must have been prescribed (or an existing medication must have been modified to treat the exacerbation),
- the episode of illness had to disrupt daily activities.

Only outpatient episodes satisfying all three criteria were included. This definition has already proven useful in earlier investigations (Marneros *et al.*, 1991b).

Episodes during the prospective follow-up period were assessed by using the Schedules for Clinical Assessment in Neuropsychiatry (SCAN).

Schedules for Clinical Assessment in Neuropsychiatry

The SCAN is a set of instruments for assessing, measuring and classifying the psychopathology and behaviour associated with major adult psychiatric disorders according to ICD-10 (van Gülick-Bailer *et al.*, 1995). SCAN consists of a Structured Clinical Interview Schedule (10th edition of PSE), a glossary of differential definitions, the Item Group Checklist and the Clinical History Schedule. In using SCAN, the interviewer decides whether a symptom was present during the specified time, as well as the degree of its severity. The SCAN interview consists of two main parts: Part 1 includes non-psychotic sections, such as physical health, worry, tension, panic, anxiety and phobias, obsessive symptoms, depressed mood, impaired thinking, concentration, energy, interests, bodily functions, weight, sleep, eating disorders, alcohol and drug abuse, and Part 2 contains sections covering psychotic and cognitive disorders and abnormalities of behaviour, speech and affect. Episodes of non-organic major affective disorder or non-organic psychotic disorder determined by use of the WHO-SCAN were included in the relapse analysis.

All interviewers were trained extensively for this instrument. Training for the WHO instrument SCAN was carried out by WHO-approved trainers, and the first ten interviews were supervised.

Diagnostic criteria

Best estimate ICD-10 diagnoses were assigned to all episodes during follow-up using all available information, including patients' reports and hospital records and SCAN interviews. Diagnoses were made according to ICD-10 research criteria (WHO, 1993). Additionally, the diagnosis 'Brief Psychosis' was made by applying the DSM-IV criteria. If information on single episodes was incomplete, the most probable diagnosis was assigned on the basis of available data.

Outcome measures

It is agreed that the outcome of psychotic disorders cannot be measured sufficiently unidimensionally, but should be described in several domains, such as symptoms, relapses, work and social adaptation. Outcome measures covering different domains often correlate, but may also dissociate in individual patients. The outcome domains are only 'loosely linked' (Strauss and Carpenter, 1972), and, as a consequence, the application of several standardised instruments describing different aspects of outcome is necessary.

The instruments used in the HASBAP were the WHO Disability Assessment Schedule (WHO/DAS), the WHO Psychological Impairments Rating Schedule (WHO/PIRS), the Global Assessment Scale (GAS) and the Positive and Negative Syndrome Scale (PANSS). The presence of residual syndromes was assessed according to the classification of Marneros and co-workers (1998). Occupational status, treatment, social mobility and other social parameters, including marriage and long-term relationships, living situation and source of income at the time of follow-up, were determined by means of a semi-structured interview.

Disability Assessment Schedule

In the HASBAP, social disability was measured using the German version of the WHO/DAS (Jung et al., 1989). This version has been developed and validated by the WHO collaborating centre in Mannheim, Germany. The WHO/DAS was conducted by means of a structured interview with the subject and one or more sources. The interview covered six domains of functioning in general behavioural domains (self-care, spare time activity, slowness, social contacts/social withdrawal, friction in interpersonal relations, emergency or crisis behaviour) and in eight domains relating to special roles (participation in household, marital role; affective, marital role; sexual, parental role, heterosexual role if single, occupational role; work performance, occupational role; interest in returning to work, general interest). In addition, a rating for global social adjustment was made (Schubart et al., 1986). All items were rated on scales ranging from 0 to 5, with higher scores designating a higher degree of handicap. In many instances, a subject did not fit into one or more particular social roles (e.g. marriage, if the subject was unmarried). In these cases, a rating of 'not applicable' was made, and no dysfunction in this area was stated. For analysis, two composite scales were used together with the global functioning scale. The composite scales 'general behaviour' and 'special roles' were generated by calculating the mean of the ratings in the according subscales. The integrated scales also ranged from 0 to 5, with higher scores designating a higher degree of handicap.

Global Assessment Scale

The level of general functioning was assessed by the widely used Global Assessment Scale (GAS, Endicott et al., 1976). The GAS is a single rating scale for evaluating the overall functioning of a subject during a specified time period on a continuum from psychiatric sickness to health. The scale values range from 1, which represents the hypothetically sickest individual, to 100, the hypothetically healthiest. In rating a particular subject, the investigators took into account both symptoms and impairments in functioning. The scale was divided into ten-point intervals each characterised by detailed anchor descriptions, but raters were encouraged to use values in-between the anchors. Rating usually (as in this study) refers to the previous week. Psychometric properties of the scale have been comprehensively evaluated (Endicott *et al.*, 1976).

The GAS has been used extensively for the evaluation of course and outcome in psychiatry and has been included as an axis in DSM-III-R. Modifications of the GAS have been suggested (Goldman *et al.*, 1992; Patterson and Lee, 1995; Sartorius *et al.*, 1996), including a separation of the rating of symptoms and social impairment. However, the original scale, with its integration of the information on both the severity of psychiatric symptoms and the level of impaired behaviour and social functioning has been shown to be reliable, conceptually sound and clinically valid (Yamauchi *et al.*, 2001). Therefore, and to retain the ability to compare the results to earlier studies, the original version of the GAS (Endicott *et al.*, 1976) was used.

Psychological Impairments Rating Schedule (WHO/PIRS)

The WHO/PIRS is a rating scale that was developed as one of the principal instruments of the WHO collaborative study on impairments and disabilities associated with schizophrenic disorders (Jablensky *et al.*, 1980). It has been used in several studies, both within and outside of the WHO Mental Health Programme (Biehl *et al.*, 1989a,b). According to the International Classification of Impairments, Disabilities and Handicaps (ICIDH), impairment is defined as 'any loss or abnormality of psychological, physiological or anatomical structure or function'. Impairments have to be differentiated both from signs and symptoms of illness and from disabilities. Impairments are less disease-specific than symptoms, but more specific than disabilities. Furthermore, disabilities are more influenced by external factors than impairments.

The WHO/PIRS primarily assesses deficits in psychological function perceived during a clinical interview. Application of the WHO/PIRS does not require the performance of a particular structured interview, but rather can be combined with a sufficiently comprehensive clinical interview during which behaviour and interactions of the subject can be observed. After examining the subject, the observer rates the subject's behaviour during the interview.

The WHO/PIRS contains 75 items from 10 domains: slowness/psychic tempo, attention/withdrawal, tendency to experience fatigue, initiative, communication by facial expression, communication by body language, affect display, conversation skills, self-representation, co-operation. In addition, a rating of the global impression of the patient's personality was made. Item definitions are compatible with the PSE (Wing *et al.*, 1974). The item ratings are integrated into three scales (general score, activity/retreat, communication behaviour). Scale values range from 0 to 5, with a higher score designating a greater degree of handicap. For purposes of analysis, the mean ratings on the WHO/PIRS general scale were compared between the subgroups.

Positive and Negative Syndrome Scale (PANSS)

The PANSS is an observer rating scale that assesses present state psychopathological symptoms in psychotic disorders using 30 items with 7-point severity scales. It was originally based on the 18-item Brief Psychiatric Rating Scale (Overall and Gorham, 1962), but compared with that scale, it represents a considerable improvement in theoretical foundation, comprehensiveness and psychometric standardisation. Conceptually, it draws on the differentiation of a positive and a negative syndrome in schizophrenia (Strauss and Carpenter, 1974; Crow, 1980), arguably hypothesised to bear different aetiological, pharmacological and prognostic import (Kay *et al.*, 1989). The 30 Items of the PANSS comprise 7 items representing different aspects of the positive syndrome, 7 items representing different aspects of the negative syndrome and 16 items representing general psychopathology. The 30 items were selected taking into account (1) their compliance with the positive-negative distinction, (2) the possibility of unambiguous classification, and (3) the desire to cover diverse realms of cognitive, affective, social and communicative functioning. Every item is defined by strict operational criteria, including detailed rating instructions for every point of severity covering a range between absent and severe.

The PANSS has undergone an extensive evaluation of reliability and validity. In the original standardisation, the PANSS scales showed an interrater reliability of 0.83–0.87 and internal reliability indicated by an alpha of 0.73–0.79 (Kay *et al.*, 1989). In chronically ill patients, the test-retest reliability of the scales was established (Kay *et al.*, 1989). In large cohorts of schizophrenic patients, the validity of the PANSS were corroborated. Meaningful correlations exist between the PANSS scales and other psychometric symptom scales, as well as between PANSS scales and biographical, clinical and sociodemographical measures (Kay *et al.*, 1989). Since its introduction, the PANSS has proved its reliability and validity in numerous studies including clinical trials of pharmacological agents and clinical studies addressing issues of the nosology of psychotic disorders.

In the HASBAP, the PANSS was applied during the second follow-up interview. For analysis, the positive and negative subscales were used, as well as the composite score calculated by adding the positive, negative and general subscore.

Assessment of persisting alterations (residual syndromes)

We prefer the term *persisting alterations* and *residual syndromes*. Our experiences with long-term investigations in affective and schizoaffective and schizophrenic disorders show that what we usually call residual symptoms are not only symptoms remaining as a small part of the full psychopathological condition, but much more: one part comprises deficits caused by the illness, but there are also phobic conditions, low self-confidence, changes of social interactional patterns, psychological attitudes not belonging to the psychopathological feature of the illness and so on. Although persisting, all these phenomena are not only residual, but also new productions (Marneros *et al.*, 1988c, 1990c, 1991b, 1998; Marneros and Rohde, 1997).

The existence of persisting alterations (residual syndromes) at follow-up was assessed using a method described by Marneros and his colleagues (Marneros *et al.*, 1991b, 1998; Marneros and Rohde, 1997): Psychopathological symptoms, as assessed during the interview, information gathered with the standardised instruments, and the observed interactional atmosphere, were integrated to draw up a phenomenological profile of the patient. Eight typologically defined types of persisting alteration were discerned, including depletion syndrome, apathetic-paranoid syndrome, adynamic deficiency syndrome, chronic psychosis, structural deformation, slight asthenic insufficiency syndrome, chronic subdepressive syndrome and chronic hyperthymic syndrome (Table 3.4). Detailed descriptions are given elsewhere (Marneros and Rohde, 1997; Marneros *et al.*, 1998). The reliability of this procedure has been demonstrated (see Table 3.5). Different profiles of persisting alterations have been shown in schizophrenic, schizoaffective and affective psychoses (Marneros *et al.*, 1991b, 1998).

Self-rating instrument: NEO-FFI

During the first follow-up interview, subjects were asked to complete the NEO Five-Factor Inventory (Costa and McCrae, 1992), a self-report questionnaire consisting of 60 questions designed to assess traits dimensionally in the five domains of neuroticism, extroversion, openness to experience, agreeableness and conscientiousness. The NEO-FFI is a widely accepted instrument to measure personality traits based on the five-factor model of personality. It has been used extensively to study personality traits in normal adults. Significant correlations have been found between self-rating in the NEO-FFI and the rating of personality traits by significant others (McCrae and Costa, 1990). The use of the NEO-FFI in psychiatric populations has been shown to be feasible, both for patients with affective disorders (Blöink *et al.*, 2004) and for patients with schizophrenia (Kentros *et al.*, 1997; Gurrera *et al.*, 2000). In the HASBAP, however, care was taken to exclude patients who were unable to complete the NEO-FFI due to cognitive deficits. The German

Table 3.4. Phenomenological constellations of persisting alterations (Marneros *et al.*, 1991b, 1998)

Depletion syndrome
– Severe reduction of drive
– Severe deficiency of energy and initiative
– Affective flattening
– Reduction of facial expressions and gestures
– 'Cool isolation'
– Severe reduction of concentration capacity
– Increased distractibility
– Patients are not aware of their disturbances
– No persisting productive psychotic symptoms

Adynamic-deficient syndrome
– Moderate reduction of the mental energetic potential
– Reduction of interest for everyday events
– Affectivity reduced, but not flattened
– Limited variation of behaviour and expression
– No 'cool isolation'
– No continuous depressive or euphoric mood
– Productive psychotic symptoms only transient and not impressive

Structural deformation of personality
– Persisting deformation of the personality
– Productive psychotic symptoms only transient and not impressive
– No severe disturbances of affectivity
– No slowness

Chronic subdepressive syndrome
– Chronic subdepressive symptoms
– No affective flattening
– No productive psychotic symptomatology
– No slowness

Apathetic-paranoid syndrome (resp. apathetic-hallucinatory syndrome)
– Persisting delusions and/or hallucinations
– Severe slowness
– Affective flattening
– Severe social withdrawal
– Loss of interest for almost all activities
– Severe reduction of energy and initiative
– Patients are not aware of their disturbances

Chronic psychosis
– Chronic productive psychotic symptomatology (in most cases paranoid symptomatology)
– No severe disturbances of affectivity, possibly slight fluctuations of mood
– No severe disturbances of expression and contact

Slight asthenic-insufficiency syndrome
– Slight reduction of mental energetic potential
– Possibility of slight, subjective perceived impairments of concentration capacity
– Slight mood disturbances
– No productive psychotic symptoms or only transient and not impressive

Chronic hyperthymic syndrome
– Chronic hyperthymic symptomatology
– No affective flattening
– No productive psychotic symptomatology
– No slowness

Table 3.5. Inter-rater reliability of the basic outcome variables

Variable	n	Parameter	Value
Outpatient psychiatric treatment	15	kappa[a]	1.00
Psychotherapy	15	kappa[a]	1.00
Suicidal behaviour during follow-up	15	kappa[a]	1.00
On psychiatric medication	15	kappa[a]	1.00
Employed	15	kappa[a]	1.00
Disability pension	15	kappa[a]	0.83
Stable heterosexual relationship	15	kappa[a]	0.90
Full autarky	15	kappa[a]	1.00
Persisting alterations	14	kappa[a]	0.66
WHO/DAS General Behaviour Subscale	14	ICC[b]	0.95
WHO/DAS Special Roles Subscale	14	ICC[b]	0.91
WHO/DAS Global Score	14	ICC[b]	0.94
PANSS Positive Subscale	14	ICC[b]	0.93
PANSS Negative Subscale	14	ICC[b]	0.94
PANSS General Subscale	14	ICC[b]	0.96
PANSS Total Scale	14	ICC[b]	0.99
GAS Global Assessment Score	14	ICC[b]	0.86

[a] kappa = Cohen's kappa.
[b] ICC = Intra-Class Correlation.

version of the NEO-FFI was employed, translated and validated by Borkenau and Ostendorf (1993).

Reliability tests

Reliability estimates for the basic outcome variables (i.e. WHO/DAS, WHO/PIRS, GAS, PANSS) were obtained. For this purpose, 15 interviews were double-coded by two raters (interviewer–observer method). Kappa values for categorical items exceeded 0.80 for nearly all items, and agreement showed a kappa of 0.65 for 'persisting alterations', which can be considered substantial (Landis and Koch, 1977). For quantitative outcome scales, intra-class correlation coefficients were excellent, ranging from 0.86 to 0.99 (Table 3.5).

Data analysis

Statistical analyses were performed using the Statistical Package for Social Sciences (SPSS), version 9.0. The primary intention was to compare the index sample of patients with ATPD with the two clinical control groups and, where this was meaningful, with the mentally healthy controls. Since there were 3–4 matched groups to compare with each other, and since, due to the comprehensive character of the study, numerous variables were assessed, the number of possible comparisons was very large. A statistical correction for multiple comparisons would have greatly diminished the statistical power, in particular with regard to the limited number of subjects. Therefore, for categorical data, generally the uncorrected significance of group comparisons was reported. Contingency tables of categorical data were analysed with χ^2 tests or Fisher's exact test as appropriate. For continuous data, where statistical power is somewhat higher, generally an analysis of variance (ANOVA) was performed with *post hoc* tests using the Scheffé procedure. This resulted in a more conservative estimation of significant differences. The statistical analysis chosen was also compatible with the character of the HASBAP, which was exploratory, rather than confirmatory. In some instances additional statistical procedures were employed. Details on these procedures are given in the appropriate sections. The level of significance was generally set at 0.05.

4

Frequency and sociobiographic characteristics of acute and transient psychotic disorders (ATPD) and brief psychoses (BP)

The frequency of ATPD

As already pointed out, there are virtually no sound epidemiological studies regarding the frequency of ATPD or BP. Susser and co-workers (1994), in their re-analysis of the DOSMED data, determined the annual incidence per 10 000 people of Non-affective Acute Remitting Psychosis (NARP) to be 0.486 for males and 0.878 for females in the developing country setting and 0.040 for males and 0.104 for females in the industrialised country setting. This compared to an annual incidence of ICD-9 schizophrenia (NARP excluded) of 1.328 for males and 1.089 for females in the developing country setting and 1.190 for males and 0.880 for females in the industrialised country setting. These data cannot be extended easily to ATPD and BP since definitions differ. The ten-fold higher incidence of NARP in the developing countries, however, corroborates the long-held impression that Brief and Acute Psychoses are much more frequent in developing than in industrialised countries.

Compared with epidemiological incidence data, it is much more feasible to determine the frequency of Brief and Acute Psychoses as the proportion of inpatients with broad definition psychotic disorders in a particular institution. Such data are available for NARP and for DSM-IV BP in the Suffolk County Mental Health project. In an analysis of 221 first-episode patients with DSM-III-R affective or non-affective psychoses including 117 cases of non-affective psychoses, Susser and co-workers (1995a) identified 7 patients with Acute Brief Psychoses (synonymous with Susser's definition of NARP as discussed above). This amounts to 3% of the whole sample or to 6% of the subsample with non-affective psychotic disorders. Another analysis from the project (Schwartz et al., 2000) relying on a larger sample found 11 patients with DSM-IV BP among 547 patients with affective or non-affective psychotic disorders (2%). Again, the proportion is higher when related only to patients with non-affective psychoses (11 of 234, 4.7%) (recalculated from Table 1 in Schwartz et al., 2000). It must be noted, however, that when diagnoses were re-evaluated

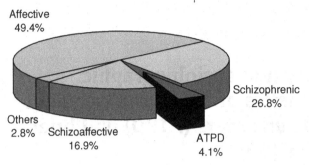

Fig. 4.1.   Proportion of Acute and Transient Psychotic Disorders (ATPD, ICD-10) in all non-organic psychotic and non-organic major affective disorders (ICD-10 F2, F3) during the period of recruitment at Martin Luther University 1993–97.

at 24 months, only 3 patients still received a diagnosis of BP (Schwartz *et al.*, 2000).

Somewhat exceptional are the data from a first-episode sample of 168 patients with broad definition psychotic disorders in Nottingham (Brewin *et al.*, 1997; Amin *et al.*, 1999). In this cohort, a diagnosis of ATPD according to ICD-10 research criteria was made in 32 patients (19% of the whole cohort). This amounts to 28% of all 113 patients with non-organic, non-affective psychotic disorders (recalculated from Table 1 in Brewin *et al.*, 1997)! In their paper, the authors compared their data with DOSMED data collected earlier in Nottingham and speculated that there might be a declining incidence of narrowly defined schizophrenia. However, the sample was also quite atypical in other respects: ATPD was diagnosed nearly twice as often in males as in females, while Mania was diagnosed much more frequently in female than in male patients. Moreover, at the three-year follow-up, only 11 patients still received a diagnosis of ATPD (Amin *et al.*, 1999).

The HASBAP was not an epidemiological study, but a clinical one. Nevertheless, it can be assumed to be fairly representative of the frequency of ATPD, as well as BP. ATPD and BP are acute and usually dramatic psychotic states that almost invariably lead to inpatient treatment. Taking into account the German health care system, it could be assumed that virtually all patients having an acute psychosis would be treated in a psychiatric hospital.

During the recruitment period (1993–1997), 1036 patients from the Psychiatric Department of Martin Luther University Hospital were diagnosed as having non-organic psychotic or non-organic affective disorders (ICD-10 categories F2 and F3); 4.1% of these patients were diagnosed as ATPD (Fig. 4.1). If only the non-organic psychotic disorders are considered (excluding the non-organic major affective disorders), then the proportion of ATPD was 8.5% (Fig. 4.2). Allocating the ATPD to the four ICD-10 subcategories already

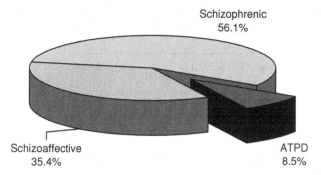

Fig. 4.2.   Proportion of Acute and Transient Psychotic Disorders (ATPD) in all non-organic psychotic disorders (ICD-10 F2) at Martin Luther University 1993–97.

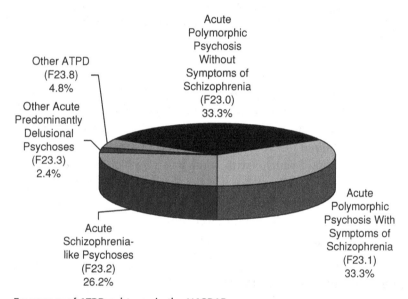

Fig. 4.3.   Frequency of ATPD subtypes in the HASBAP.

mentioned, namely:

- 'Acute Polymorphic Psychoses' (F23.0/1),
- 'Acute Schizophrenia-like Psychoses' (F23.2),
- 'Other Acute Predominantly Delusional Psychoses' (F23.3) and
- 'Other Acute and Transient Psychoses' (F23.8)

it was found that two-thirds of the patients (67%) could be allocated to the sub-category 'Acute Polymorphic Psychoses' (Fig. 4.3 and Table 4.1). In other words, the vast majority of ATPD had a polymorphous symptomatology. The ICD-10 placed the polymorphous subtype in two categories; namely, in the 'Acute

Table 4.1. Frequency of subtypes of ATPD according to ICD-10

	n	%
Acute Polymorphic Psychoses (F23.0/F23.1)	28	67
Acute Schizophrenia-like Psychoses (F23.2)	11	26
Other Acute Predominantly Delusional Psychoses (F23.3)	1	2
Other Acute and Transient Psychoses (F23.8)	2	5

Table 4.2. Frequency of Subtypes of Acute Polymorphic Psychoses according to ICD-10

Acute Polymorphic Psychosis	n	%[a]
... Without Symptoms of Schizophrenia (F23.0)	14	50
... With Symptoms of Schizophrenia (F23.1)	14	50

[a] Per cent of all patients with Acute Polymorphic Psychoses.

Polymorphic Psychotic Disorders *Without* Symptoms of schizophrenia' (F23.0) category and the 'Acute Polymorphic Psychotic Disorders *With* Symptoms of Schizophrenia' (F23.1) category. In the HASBAP population, it emerged that exactly one-half of the polymorphous group displayed schizophrenic symptoms, and the other half did not (Table 4.2). In the sample of Jørgensen and co-workers (1996) the proportion of patients with Acute Polymorphic Psychoses was nearly identical (35/51, 69%), although only 25% of the Polymorphic Psychoses also showed symptoms of schizophrenia (7 of 28). In the study of Das and co-workers (1999), again 62.5% of the ATPD sample were Acute Polymorphic Psychoses, and 19% of these had symptoms of schizophrenia.

Frequency of DSM-IV Brief Psychoses

By definition, the DSM-IV diagnosis 'Brief Psychosis' is much more narrow than the ICD-10 diagnosis 'Acute and Transient Psychotic Disorder' (see p. 12). As a consequence, all patients diagnosed as having DSM-IV diagnosis 'Brief Psychosis' also have an ICD-10 diagnosis ATPD; whereas not all ATPD patients also have a 'Brief Psychosis', according to DSM-IV. The HASBAP found that 26 patients (61.9% of those with ATPD) could be diagnosed as having a DSM-IV diagnosis 'Brief Psychosis' and 31% of the patients with ATPD fulfilled the DSM-IV criteria of 'Schizophreniform Disorder' (295.40) (see Table 4.3). The proportion of DSM-IV 'Brief Psychosis' within the population of non-organic psychotic and non-organic affective disorders of the investigated period was only 2.5% (Fig. 4.4). This finding confirms the assumption of DSM-IV authors that Brief Psychoses

Table 4.3. Diagnoses of patients with ICD-10 ATPD according to DSM-IV

Diagnosis according to DSM-IV	n	%
Brief Psychotic Disorder 298.8	26	61.9
Schizophreniform Disorder 295.40	13	31.0
Psychotic Disorder NOS 298.9	2	4.8
Delusional Disorder 297.1	1	2.4

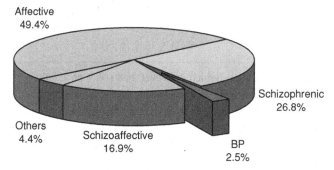

Fig. 4.4.   Proportion of Brief Psychotic Disorders (DSM-IV, BP) in all non-organic psychotic and non-organic major affective episodes at Martin Luther University 1993–97.

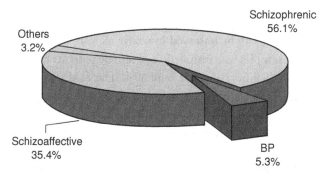

Fig. 4.5.   Proportion of Brief Psychotic Disorders (DSM-IV) in all non-organic psychotic episodes at Martin Luther University 1993–97.

as defined by DSM-IV are not very frequent (APA, 1994). The proportion of the DSM-IV diagnoses 'Brief Psychosis' among the group of non-organic psychotic disorders is approximately 5% (see Fig. 4.5). The remaining patients in the ATPD group were distributed over the DSM-IV categories 'Schizophreniform Disorder' (31%), 'Delusional Disorder' (2.4%) and 'Psychotic Disorder Not Otherwise Specified'

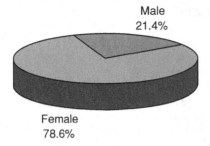

Male
21.4%

Female
78.6%

Fig. 4.6.   Gender distribution in patients with ATPD.

(4.8%) (Table 4.3). The concordance of ATPD and BP has already been considered above (see p. 14).

> Conclusion: With one exception (which, however, has some peculiarities), studies in industrialised countries indicate that Brief and Acute Psychoses are infrequent disorders that comprise about 5–10% of all inpatients with non-organic, non-affective psychotic disorders. The frequency is lower when more restricted criteria are used for diagnosis as in DSM-IV BP. The frequency of Brief and Acute Psychoses is considerably higher in developing countries.
>   It emerges as a stable finding that about 2/3 of all patients with Acute and Transient Psychoses can be classified as belonging to the Polymorphic subtype.

Gender distribution

A female preponderance can be observed in nearly all samples of Brief and Acute Psychoses. In ATPD samples, the proportion of female patients has been reported at 76% (1996), 71.1% (Sajith *et al.*, 2002) and 60% (Das *et al.*, 1999). Studies using varying definitions of Non-affective Acute Remitting Psychoses included between 57% (Susser and Wanderling, 1994) and 86% (Susser *et al.*, 1995a) female patients. No information on gender is available for the 11 patients with DSM-IV BP of Schwartz and co-workers (2000). The only exception to female preponderance is the Nottingham study of Brewin and co-workers (1997), with 66% males among 32 patients with ATPD, but this sample seems to be atypical also in regard to the relative frequency of ATPD and schizophrenia.

In the HASBAP, the vast majority (78.6%) of patients diagnosed as having an ATPD were female (Fig. 4.6). This corresponds to a female:male ratio of 3.7:1. Female preponderance was particularly striking when compared to gender distribution in the other diagnostic groups. For comparison, Fig. 4.7 gives the gender distribution for all patients treated as inpatients at the same institution during the period from 1993 to 1997 for non-organic psychotic disorders or non-organic major

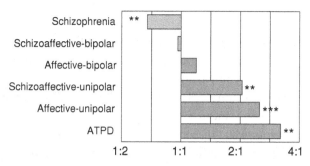

Fig. 4.7.   Gender distribution according to diagnostic category in all non-organic psychotic and non-organic major affective disorders (ICD-10 F2, F3) during the period of investigation at Martin Luther University 1993–97 ($n = 1036$ inpatients). Significance of deviation from equal distribution: **$P < 0.01$, ***$P < 0.001$.

affective disorders. Although an inpatient population may show selection bias and is not identical with the whole population suffering from a psychotic disorder, the gender distributions found are very similar to gender ratios reported in epidemiological studies (Leung and Chue, 2000). The remarkable predominance of females in the group of ATPD with a female:male ratio of 3.7:1 is one of the most important findings of the HASBAP. This overrepresentation of female patients is in accordance with the findings of other studies on Brief and Acute Psychoses as reported above. Even before the definition of ATPD and BP, brief psychotic disorders with a favourable prognosis have generally been observed to occur preferentially in female patients (Ring *et al.*, 1991; Susser *et al.*, 1995a).

The uneven gender distribution is an argument which perhaps could provide evidence for the validity of a delineation of ATPD from schizophrenia, which is equally prevalent in both genders (Dohrenwend and Dohrenwend, 1976; WHO, 1979; Munk-Jørgensen, 1985; Schubart, 1986; Möller and von Zerssen, 1986; Häfner, 1987; Lewine, 1988; Marneros *et al.*, 1991b; Leung and Chue, 2000). Nevertheless, for such a delineation more factors are necessary than gender distribution.

In Bipolar Schizoaffective Disorders, there is also an equal distribution among females and males (Marneros *et al.*, 1989a, 1990a, 1990b, 1991b). The differences in gender ratio between ATPD and Bipolar Schizoaffective Disorders are also a finding that could support a distinction between the two psychotic disorders in the same way as mentioned above.

> Conclusion: Acute and Transient Psychotic Disorders are much more frequent in women than in men. This constitutes an important difference to schizophrenia and to schizoaffective disorders.

Age at onset

Data on the age at onset of psychotic disorders are difficult to compare across studies if the exact demographic distribution of the population is not known. This is especially important for comparisons between industrialised and developing countries. Among the studies on ATPD, the two studies from India reported an age at onset of 26.9 ± 10.9 years (mean ± SD) (Sajith *et al.*, 2002) and 25 ± 9.4 years (Das *et al.*, 1999), respectively. In contrast, the patients in the Danish study of Jørgensen and co-workers (1996) had a mean age at onset of 33 years (range 18–65 years). These differences may well represent differences in the age distribution of the general populations.

More information can be gained if the age at onset is compared between different diagnoses in patients drawn from the same population. In the re-analysis of DOSMED data by Susser and co-workers (1994), age at onset data are reported separately according to gender, setting (developing country vs. industrialised country) and diagnosis (NARP vs. other cases of schizophrenia). In this analysis, age at onset in males was similar for NARP and other ICD-9 schizophrenia (22.4 vs. 23.0 years in the developing country setting; 25.5 vs. 26.0 years in the industrialised country setting). For female patients, age at onset was somewhat lower in patients with NARP than in patients with schizophrenia (22.4 vs. 25.7 years in the developing country setting; 24.9 vs. 30.7 years in the industrialised country setting).

The data of the HASBAP allowed a comparison between ATPD patients and the clinical control groups which were drawn from the same population. In these samples, there were no differences regarding age at onset between ATPD patients (mean 35.7 years) and patients with 'Positive Schizophrenia' (mean 35.3 years). Marked differences emerged, however, between ATPD and patients with Bipolar Schizoaffective Psychosis, who experienced their onset at a significantly earlier age (mean 28.6 years). More than one-half of the patients with ATPD became ill after the age of 33 years, while for the patients with BSAD, the median age at onset was found to be 24.7 years (Table 4.4). Although the first manifestation of the illness is possible in every age for all three diagnostic groups, it seems that after an age of 50, it is rare, especially in the group of BSAD, but also for ATPD (Table 4.4, Fig. 4.8). It is also interesting that the onset of the illness before the twentieth year of life occurred in only one patient with ATPD, but in 26% of the patients with Bipolar Schizoaffective Disorder.

There were large and consistent gender differences in age at onset for all three clinical groups with male patients falling ill at a younger age than female patients (age at onset for female vs. male patients in ATPD 37.1 ± 11.7 vs. 30.8 ± 7.3 years; in PS 38.0 ± 14.4 vs. 25.5 ± 5.2 years; in BSAD 30.0 ± 11.6 vs. 23.4 ± 4.7 years). An

Table 4.4. Age at onset

	ATPD $n = 42$	PS $n = 42$	BSAD $n = 42$	
	n (%)	n (%)	n (%)	Statistical analysis[a]
10 to 19 years	1 (2.4)	4 (9.5)	11 (26.2)	
20 to 29 years	14 (33.3)	16 (38.1)	15 (35.7)	
30 to 39 years	15 (35.7)	8 (19.0)	9 (21.4)	
40 to 49 years	9 (21.4)	7 (16.7)	6 (14.3)	
50 to 59 years	1 (2.4)	4 (9.5)	0	
60 to 69 years	1 (2.4)	2 (4.8)	1 (2.4)	
70 to 79 years	1 (2.4)	1 (2.4)	0	
Mean	35.8	35.3	28.6	$P = 0.011$
Standard deviation	11.1	13.9	10.8	ATPD > BSAD*
Median	33.5	31.1	24.7	PS > BSAD*
Range	18–70	16–73	15–61	

[a] ANOVA, *post hoc* comparisons significant in Scheffé's procedure are indicated; * $P < 0.05$.

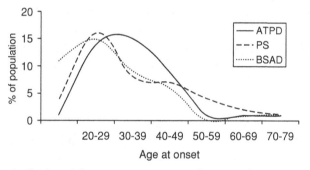

Fig. 4.8.   Distribution of the age at onset (age at first episode) in 42 patients with ATPD, 42 controls with PS and 42 controls with BSAD.

overall analysis of variance with age at onset as the dependent variable and gender and diagnosis as fixed factors yielded a highly significant influence of gender ($F = 11.384$, d.f. $= 1$, $P = 0.001$) and a marginal influence of diagnosis ($F = 2.909$, d.f. $= 1$, $P = 0.057$), while the interaction of gender and diagnosis was insignificant. This finding of a marked gender difference in age at onset for ATPD as well as for schizophrenia contradicts the findings of Susser and co-workers (1994). In their study of NARP, these authors found a lacking gender difference in age at onset and argued that this finding supported the nosological independence of NARP. Overall, the findings of the HASBAP do not support the notion that ATPD is essentially a disease of young people. On the contrary, ATPD could occur at practically every age and the mean age at onset tended to be higher than the age at onset in epidemiological samples with schizophrenia. However, the fact that there was no significant difference between ATPD and Positive Schizophrenia in the HASBAP is most probably due to a methodological artefact. Data reported in the literature support a significantly lower age at onset of schizophrenia than that found in the HASBAP (WHO, 1979; Loranger, 1984; Möller and von Zerssen, 1986; Schubart, 1986; Lewine, 1988; Bardenstein and McGlashan, 1990; Marneros et al., 1991b; Tsuang et al., 1995; Häfner and an der Heiden, 1997; Häfner et al., 1998).

A possible explanation for the finding regarding the age at onset of schizophrenia is that, due to the case-control design of the HASBAP, the group was not representative for patients with schizophrenia in general but was highly selected. Two features of the sample were associated with higher age at onset, namely the feature 'Positive Schizophrenia' and the feature 'female predominance' (WHO, 1979; Schubart, 1986; Lewine, 1988; Marneros et al., 1991b; Tsuang et al., 1995; Häfner and an der Heiden, 1997; Häfner et al., 1998). In addition, although controls were not directly matched to age at onset, age at index episode and age at onset were highly correlated in the HASBAP sample, in particular for patients with PS (Pearson's r for the correlation of age at first episode and age at index episode: $r = 0.798$, $P < 0.001$ in ATPD, $r = 0.872$, $P < 0.001$ in PS, $r = 0.608$, $P < 0.001$ in BSAD). Matching the controls to the index patients for age at index episode, therefore, will make the controls more similar to the ATPD patients in age at onset as well. As a result of the matching process, existing differences in age at onset between the groups will be diluted. All this leads to the consequence that the group differences in age at onset in the HASBAP may *underestimate* the 'real' (epidemiological) differences between the diagnostic groups. While the lower age at onset of BSAD patients most probably reflects a 'true' difference, the relatively high age at onset of the PS sample is therefore probably due to a methodological artefact.

Consequently, the findings in the HASBAP regarding age at onset could be an argument supporting the delineation of ATPD from Bipolar Schizoaffective Disorders. In contrast, the lack of a difference in age at onset between ATPD and PS does not speak against the delineation of ATPD from schizophrenia. In the HASBAP, the PS control group is biased towards a later onset due to the selecting factors 'Positive Schizophrenia' and 'female predominance' and due to the matching for age at index episode. When the epidemiological literature on schizophrenia is taken into account, the age at onset of ATPD appears to be much higher than that of schizophrenia.

Conclusion: Although Acute and Transient Psychotic Disorders may occur at any age, the age at onset for Acute and Transient Psychotic Disorders seems to peak in the mid-thirties. Age at onset in Acute and Transient Psychotic Disorders therefore appears to be considerably higher than in schizophrenia. This difference in age at onset between Acute and Transient Psychotic Disorders and Bipolar Schizoaffective Disorders could also be an argument supporting the separation of the two psychotic disorders. Earlier reports that Acute and Transient Psychotic Disorders did not show the gender difference in age at onset typical for schizophrenia were not confirmed by later results.

Season of birth

A special pattern of birth rates has long been assumed to exist in psychotic patients, in particular an excess of spring and winter births in patients with schizophrenia (Barry and Barry, 1961, 1964; Torrey and Torrey, 1980; Bradbury and Miller, 1985; Häfner, 1987; Torrey and Bowler, 1990). This finding has received much attention because of its possible aetiological relevance. According to the hypothesis adhered to by most authors, viral infections during the second month of gestation, which are most prevalent during the winter months, may affect brain development (Munk-Jørgensen and Ewald, 2001). The resulting lesion would later act as an aetiological factor in the manifestation of psychosis. In the pathogenesis of schizophrenia, the viral hypothesis has not been universally accepted, but some epidemiological evidence has accumulated in favour of the hypothesis (Munk-Jørgensen and Ewald, 2001).

The season of birth might be of particular relevance for ATPD, as postulated by some authors who have investigated cycloid psychoses. Franzek and Beckmann (1992) investigated a hypothesis of Leonhard (1957) in which patients with cycloid psychoses display a more deviant seasonal birth rate pattern than patients with so-called 'unsystematic schizophrenia'. According to Leonhard, genetic, not environmental factors, play a major role in the aetiology of unsystematic schizophrenia. In contrast, cycloid psychoses (as in the so-called 'systematic' schizophrenias), show less genetic influence, but more harmful environmental factors. Analysing 1299 of Leonhard's case records, Franzek and Beckmann (1992) indeed found elevated rates of early spring births in cycloid psychoses, but not in 'unsystematic schizophrenias'. With the exception of the HASBAP, no study has so far reported season-of-birth data on ICD-10 ATPD or DSM-IV BP.

In the sample of the HASBAP, no significant difference was found regarding the season of birth between the psychotic groups, or between those groups and the mentally healthy people (Table 4.5). The small number of subjects involved,

Table 4.5. Month and season of birth

	ATPD $n = 42$	PS $n = 42$	BSAD $n = 42$	CNTR $n = 42$
Month of birth				
January	4 (9.5)	5 (11.9)	1 (2.4)	10 (23.8)
February	6 (14.3)	3 (7.1)	3 (7.1)	3 (7.1)
March	2 (4.8)	7 (16.7)	1 (2.4)	3 (7.1)
April	7 (16.7)	1 (2.4)	7 (16.7)	3 (7.1)
May	3 (7.1)	4 (9.5)	5 (11.9)	5 (11.9)
June	5 (11.9)	2 (4.8)	8 (19.0)	–
July	1 (2.4)	7 (16.7)	3 (7.1)	5 (11.9)
August	3 (7.1)	4 (9.5)	1 (2.4)	2 (4.8)
September	3 (7.1)	3 (7.1)	2 (4.8)	2 (4.8)
October	4 (9.5)	1 (2.4)	2 (4.8)	2 (4.8)
November	3 (7.1)	4 (9.5)	4 (9.5)	3 (7.1)
December	1 (2.4)	1 (2.4)	5 (11.9)	4 (9.5)
Season of birth				
Spring (March–May)	12 (28.6)	12 (28.6)	13 (31.0)	11 (26.2)
Summer (June–August)	9 (21.4)	13 (31.0)	12 (28.6)	7 (16.7)
Autumn (September–November)	10 (23.8)	8 (19.0)	8 (19.0)	7 (16.7)
Winter (December–February)	11 (26.2)	9 (21.4)	9 (21.4)	17 (40.5)

No significant differences between groups.

however, precludes a comparison of these findings with the results obtained from big epidemiological studies.

> Conclusion: There is no support for the hypothesis connecting season of birth and the aetiology of Acute and Transient Psychotic Disorders.

Broken home

A 'broken home' situation has been established as a useful concept, both in adult, as well as in child and adolescent, psychiatry (Gmur and Tschopp, 1987; Marneros *et al.*, 1990a; Sieber and Angst, 1990; Heikkinen *et al.*, 1997; Bassarath, 2001). With the exception of the HASBAP, there are no pertinent studies on ATPD. Since universally accepted criteria for the diagnosis of a 'broken home' did not exist, for the purposes of the HASBAP an operational definition was used that has proven to be reliable and practical in several earlier studies (Marneros *et al.*, 1990a, 1991b, 1994).

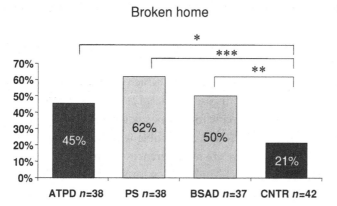

Fig. 4.9.   Frequency of a broken home situation. *$P < 0.05$, **$P < 0.01$, ***$P < 0.001$.

'Broken home' was defined as a situation in which, before the age of 15 years, at least one of the following criteria was fulfilled:

- death or loss of one or both parents,
- separation or divorce of the parents,
- growing up without natural parents,
- growing up in a foster home or an equivalent institution,
- growing up without one parent,
- severe addiction of one or both parents.

Using this definition, it was found that a high number of patients in all diagnostic groups had a broken home situation: the number of patients with a broken home situation was 19 (45.2%) in ATPD patients, 26 (61.9%) in PS patients and 21 (50%) in BSAD patients. In the mentally healthy controls, the frequency of a broken home situation was much lower (9 subjects, 21.4%). The differences between each of the diagnostic groups and the mentally healthy control group were statistically significant, while the differences between the psychiatric groups were not (Fig. 4.9). This data suggested that a broken home situation was related to all three psychotic disorders, without differences among them. The findings are in agreement with the present state of knowledge: as studies from different fields of psychiatry have shown, elevated rates of 'broken home' are not only found in psychotic and affective disorders (Angst, 1966; Bleuler, 1972; Stastny et al., 1984; Gmur and Tschopp, 1987; Akiskal, 1989; Marneros et al., 1990a), but also in conduct disorder (Bassarath, 2001), substance abuse (Sieber and Angst, 1990), borderline personality disorder (Snyder et al., 1985), suicide (Goldney, 1981) and in forensic populations (Offord et al., 1979; Marneros et al., 1994; Berger et al., 1999).

A broken home situation thus appears to have a general and unspecific relevance to the occurrence of major mental disorders, but not a specific relevance. The pathogenetic mechanisms by which a broken home constellation may influence the development and course of disease are largely unknown. In recent years, animal models showing that early parental loss can lead to lasting neuronal alterations in the developing brain have found increased interest. These findings indicate a possible pathogenetic mechanism through which parental loss may contribute to the vulnerability to psychiatric disease (Agid *et al.*, 1999). Again, however, this mechanism does not seem to be specific for any nosological entity (Agid *et al.*, 1999).

The findings of the HASBAP are compatible with the findings of the Cologne Study, which showed that there are no differences regarding the frequency of broken home situations among schizophrenic, schizoaffective and affective disorders (Marneros *et al.*, 1991b). However, in the clinical groups of the HASBAP, the frequency of broken home situations was markedly higher than that found in the Cologne Study, where 25.5–36.6% of the patients fulfilled the criteria of a 'broken home'. There is no full explanation for this difference, although regional and cohort effects are probably implicated. Divorce rates in the former German Democratic Republic (East Germany) have been considerably higher than in the Federal Republic of Germany (West Germany). While this fact may explain a part of the difference between the HASBAP and the Cologne study, it does not affect the differences between clinical groups and mentally healthy controls, who grew up in the same society. The discussion of the findings on 'broken home', thus emphasises the methodological utility of a case-control design as adopted in the HASBAP.

> Conclusion: A broken home situation can be found significantly more frequently in all three psychotic groups (Acute and Transient Psychotic Disorders, Positive Schizophrenia, Bipolar Schizoaffective Disorder) in comparison to mentally healthy people, but there is no difference between the types of psychoses.

Mental disorders in the family

With the exception of the investigation of Das and co-workers (1999, see below), family studies exclusively concerning Brief Psychoses, especially ATPD, have not been systematically carried out. Findings regarding so-called cycloid psychoses (von Trostorff, 1968; Perris, 1974; Ungvari, 1985; Maj, 1990b; Franzek and Beckmann, 1998a, 1998b), bouffée délirante (Maj, 1989, 1990b) or 'atypical psychosis' (McCabe and Strömgren, 1975; McCabe and Cadoret, 1976) cannot be extended to ATPD or BP without problems. The groups of the above-mentioned disorders are not identical with ATPD.

Those family studies that used DSM or ICD criteria mostly focused on the 'major' categories, namely schizophrenia and affective disorder. A notable exception is the

Roscommon Family Study (Kendler *et al.*, 1993b, 1993a). In this study, patients and relatives of patients were investigated according to DSM-III-R criteria. The categories 'schizophreniform', 'delusional' and 'atypical psychotic disorders' were combined into the category 'Other Non-affective Psychoses' (ONAP). This category could be partially equivalent to ATPD. Patients diagnosed as having ONAP more frequently (with significance) had schizophrenic relatives, and also (without significance) more relatives with schizoaffective disorders and ONAP. Thus, the Roscommon Family Study supports the idea of a spectrum concept, but not of a separate nosological entity of a 'non-affective non-schizophrenic psychosis' (Kendler and Walsh, 1995).

The only family study on patients with ICD-10 ATPD was conducted in Chandigarh/India by Das and co-workers (1999). The authors recruited 40 probands with ATPD and 40 schizophrenic control probands. Seventy-five per cent of all living first-degree relatives between the ages of 15 and 45 years could be personally interviewed. The investigators found a 3.35 times higher morbid risk for ATPD in relatives of ATPD probands than in relatives of probands with schizophrenia. They also found a 4.5 times higher morbid risk for schizophrenia in relatives of probands with schizophrenia than in relatives of probands with ATPD. The overall morbid risk was 8.99 in relatives of probands with schizophrenia, and 4.60 in relatives of probands with ATPD (recalculated from Table 3 of Das *et al.*, 1999).

In the HASBAP, a detailed family history for each subject was obtained using all available information, including the subjects' own reports and information from the case records. As explained above (p. 60), no face-to-face interviews with the relatives were conducted. With respect to the limited nature of the information available on the secondary cases, and to avoid 'false diagnoses', broad diagnostic categories were created. The category 'psychotic disorders' includes schizophrenia, schizoaffective and other psychotic disorders including Brief Psychoses (characterised by delusions or hallucinations). The category 'major affective disorders' included all major affective (manic or depressive) disorders. The category 'psychotic or major affective disorders' includes the former two categories and all relatives who probably suffered from a major affective or psychotic disorder, but in whom a differential diagnosis was not possible due to insufficient data. The category 'alcohol abuse' included all relatives with clinically relevant abuse or dependency. The category 'any mental disorders' comprised all above-mentioned categories and all other relevant psychiatric disorders. For comparison with other studies, data on morbid risk corrected by the age and number of first-degree relatives were reported according to the method proposed by Weinberg (Faraone *et al.*, 1999). As the risk period, the age range from 18 to 60 years was defined.

The results of this analysis are given in Table 4.6. Rates for 'any mental disorder' were increased in all clinical groups in comparison to the mentally healthy controls

Table 4.6. Mental disorders in the family (number and proportion of affected first-degree relatives, morbid risk calculated with Weinberg correction)

	Diagnosis of the index proband				
	ATPD	PS	BSAD	CNTR	Statistical analysis[a]
Number of first-degree relatives with sufficient information	198	186	209	247	
Corrected number of relatives[b]	118.5	103.0	127.0	139.5	
Relatives with any mental disorder[c]	24 (20.3)	28 (27.2)	22 (17.3)	5 (3.6)	ATPD > CNTR*** PS > CNTR*** BSAD > CNTR***
Relatives with psychotic disorders[c]	4 (3.4)	5 (4.9)	1 (0.8)	1 (0.7)	n.s.
Relatives with major affective disorders[c]	3 (2.5)	0	6 (4.7)	0	BSAD > CNTR* BSAD > PS*
Relatives with psychotic or major affective disorder[c,d]	8 (6.8)	8 (7.8)	11 (8.7)	1 (0.7)	ATPD > CNTR* PS > CNTR** BSAD > CNTR**
Relatives with alcohol abuse[c]	7 (5.9)	6 (5.8)	2 (1.6)	1 (0.7)	ATPD > CNTR* PS > CNTR*

[a] Only pairwise comparisons significant in χ^2 test or Fisher's exact test are shown. * $P < 0.05$, ** $P < 0.01$, *** $P < 0.001$, n.s. no significance.

[b] Calculated according to the method of Weinberg with an assumed period of risk from age 18–60 years.

[c] n (Morbid risk in %).

[d] Includes relatives with psychotic or major affective disorder (no differentiation possible).

(the relative morbid risk for ATPD was 5.6, the risk for PS was 7.8, and the risk for BSAD was 4.8). The differences between the clinical groups and the healthy controls were all highly significant. There was also a significantly higher incidence of any mental disorder in relatives of PS patients when compared to relatives of BSAD patients.

Rates for the broad category of psychotic or major affective disorders were also increased (relative morbid risk for ATPD was 9.7, the risk for PS was 11.1 and the risk for BSAD was 12.3). While the differences between the clinical groups and the healthy controls were all significant, no significant differences were found among the clinical groups.

The rates of major affective and psychotic disorders were also considered separately, disregarding all cases in which no reasonable differential diagnosis was possible on the basis of the available information. In ATPD, almost equal numbers of relatives with psychotic ($n = 4$) and affective disorders ($n = 3$) were found. In PS, in all relatives with sufficient information, the illness was psychotic ($n = 5$), no definite major affective illness were found. In BSAD, the majority of secondary cases were affective ($n = 5$) and only one psychotic. However, due to the small number of subjects in each category, the only significant differences were a higher number of relatives with affective disorders in BSAD than in patients with schizophrenia and in mentally healthy controls.

Rates for alcohol abuse were significantly elevated only for relatives of ATPD and PS patients (the relative morbid risk was 8.4 for ATPD and 8.3 for PS). The data on alcohol abuse, however, has to be interpreted with great reservation, because the numbers in this category are very small and the problem of underreporting, which is inherent to the family history design, might have been particularly important in this category. The data of the HASBAP can only with limitations be compared to studies involving direct examination of relatives. Nevertheless, the morbid risks for major affective or psychotic disorder in the HASBAP were similar to the values given by Das and co-workers (1999), where a morbid risk of 4.60 for relatives of ATPD patients and one of 8.99 for relatives of patients with schizophrenia (see above) were found. The frequency of affective disorders was higher in the HASBAP than in the study of Das and co-workers (1999). A reliable differentiation between ATPD and schizophrenia in the relatives was not possible. As already discussed, a more detailed diagnostic analysis of the secondary cases would have been desirable, but is not possible from the HASBAP data.

Conclusion: The rate of psychotic and major affective disorders in first-degree relatives of Acute and Transient Psychotic Disorders patients is increased to a similar degree as in the relatives of patients with Positive Schizophrenia and Bipolar Schizoaffective Disorder. There is some indication that, in relatives of patients with Acute and Transient Psychotic Disorder, rates of both affective and psychotic disorders are elevated. In contrast, secondary cases in Positive Schizophrenia are mostly psychotic, and in Bipolar Schizoaffective Disorder, secondary cases are mostly affective. This finding might support a connection between Acute and Transient Psychotic Disorders and affective disorders. However, these results are only tentative and need replication by studies involving direct investigation of relatives.

Educational level

The level of education, as determined by the amount and type of schooling received, is a parameter that can be readily and reliably assessed. Problems might arise in comparing the results of different studies because the educational systems – as is well known – vary between different countries, even among the European countries. In the study of Das and co-workers (1999), which compared 40 patients with ATPD and 40 patients with schizophrenia, educational achievement was dichotomised in 'above high school' and 'below and up to high school'. In this sample, more than half of the ATPD patients ($n = 23$), but only slightly more than one-third of the patients with schizophrenia ($n = 14$), had education above high school level. The difference was statistically significant. The other Indian study investigating 45 patients with Acute Polymorphic Psychosis comprised subjects of much lower education: 47% of this sample were illiterate and only 20% achieved college education. There was no comparison group. The low level of schooling might, however, be characteristic for the area the study patients were recruited (Sajith *et al.*, 2002).

When classifying the patients of the HASBAP according to educational achievement, it has to be considered that the majority of subjects grew up in the former German Democratic Republic (East Germany), which had a different educational system then the Federal Republic of Germany (West Germany). It was therefore decided to disregard school type (as long as the subjects attended a regular school) and to classify the level of education according to the highest grade in school successfully completed. The feature 'education' was coded in four categories: 'very low level', 'low level', 'medium level' and 'high level'. A *high level* of education was defined as completion of the 12th grade. A *medium level* of education was defined as completion of the 10th grade and a *low level* of education was defined as completion of the 8th grade. Subjects with less schooling or subjects that attended a special school were assigned a *very low* level of education.

There was no significant difference between patients with ATPD and the mentally healthy group regarding educational level, although a relatively high number of patients with a very low level of education (i.e. no completion of regular school) was conspicuous (Table 4.7). In addition, patients with BSAD did not have any difference to the mentally healthy group. Interestingly, patients with a very high level of education were significantly scarce in the PS group, both when compared to ATPD and to mentally healthy controls. Although easy to assess, the interpretation of data on the level of education is not entirely straightforward. The level of education achieved may reflect different influences on individual scholastic development, including cognitive abilities, the socio-economic level of the primary family, and, possibly, early signs of a mental illness. An association of a low level of education and the development of schizophrenia has long been described (Campbell and Malone, 1991; Jones *et al.*, 1993). While some authors interpret this finding in the context of social status (Angermeyer and Klusmann, 1987; Goldstein, 1990; Aro *et al.*, 1995), there are alternative explanations. The poor performance in school of patients later diagnosed with

Table 4.7. Educational level

	ATPD $n = 42$	PS $n = 42$	BSAD $n = 42$	CNTR $n = 42$	
	n (%)	n (%)	n (%)	n (%)	Statistical analysis[a]
Very low	6 (14.3)	5 (11.9)	1 (2.4)	1 (2.4)	n.s.
Low	10 (23.8)	13 (31.0)	13 (31.0)	14 (33.3)	n.s.
Medium	16 (38.1)	22 (52.4)	22 (52.4)	18 (42.9)	n.s.
High	10 (23.8)	2 (4.8)	6 (14.3)	9 (21.4)	ATPD > PS*
					CNTR > PS*

[a] Only pairwise comparisons with significant differences (χ^2 test or Fisher's exact test, two-tailed) are shown. *$P < 0.05$, n.s. no significance.

schizophrenia may result from premorbid or preclinical abnormalities (Olin *et al.*, 1998). It may also be the consequence of subtle neuropsychiatric impairments postulated by the neurodevelopmental theory of schizophrenia (Murray, 1994).

There are also more unspecific correlations of educational underachievement and psychiatric illness. A large epidemiological study conducted in Finland showed that not attending normal class (i.e., class below age level or in special school) at the age of 14 increases the likelihood of later hospitalisation for a number of psychiatric disorders, including schizophrenia and non-schizophrenic psychotic disorders (Isohanni *et al.*, 1998). Within samples of patients with psychotic disorders, a low level of education foretells an unfavourable course (Viinamaki *et al.*, 1996; Menezes *et al.*, 1997). Schizophrenia, narrowly defined, still remains the disorder in which low educational achievement is found most consistently. This was also confirmed by the results of the Cologne Study, where patients with schizophrenia showed less educational achievement than patients with affective or schizoaffective disorders (Marneros *et al.*, 1991b).

> Conclusion: When the available evidence is evaluated, it appears that the educational level in Acute and Transient Psychotic Disorder is generally higher than in schizophrenia and indiscernible from mentally healthy controls.

Socio-economic status

The complex interaction of social class (socio-economic status, SES) and mental illness has received much attention and has given rise to controversial discussions (Eaton, 1985; Angermeyer and Klusmann, 1987). A review of the topic is beyond the scope of this book. Briefly summarised, an association of low SES and the occurrence of mental disorders is well established (Hollingshead and Redlich, 1958; Dunham, 1965; Dohrenwend *et al.*, 1992). Possible explanatory models include the theory of 'social causation' (low SES leads to mental disorder) and social selection (people with psychopathology experience a 'downward social drift'). Both theories, which are not mutually exclusive (Ritsher *et al.*, 2001), have received empirical support, but their relative importance varies by diagnosis (Dohrenwend *et al.*, 1998). For example, in the case of schizophrenia, a low socio-economic background in the primary family has been shown to be associated with an increased risk of adult-onset schizophrenia (Harrison *et al.*, 2001). On the other hand, there is evidence that patients with schizophrenia undergo a downward social drift (Eaton, 1985; Angermeyer and Klusmann, 1987; Dohrenwend *et al.*, 1992).

Both findings are in concordance with the results of the Cologne Study (Marneros *et al.*, 1991b). In the Cologne Study, schizophrenic patients more often came from a low socio-economic background than would be expected from the sociodemographic structure of the general population. This result was not true for the schizoaffective and affective patients studied (Marneros *et al.*, 1991b). Schizophrenic patients also experienced negative social mobility more often than schizoaffective and affective patients, and this social decline was present even before the onset of the disorder (Marneros *et al.*, 1991b).

Up to the HASBAP, no systematic data on socio-economic status in ATPD have been reported so far. Das and co-workers (1999), in their comparison of 40 patients with ATPD and 40 patients with schizophrenia, noted that significantly more patients with ATPD were employed than patients with schizophrenia.

The HASBAP explored whether there were differences in SES and social mobility among the clinical samples or between the clinical samples and the mentally healthy controls. The classification of socio-economic status followed the criteria of Kleining and Moore (1975a,b), who in turn largely adapted the classification of Hollingshead and Redlich (1958). It is a dilemma that this classification, developed in western societies, might not adequately reflect the social structure in the socialist economic system of the former German Democratic Republic, in which most of the subjects of the HASBAP lived from 1949–1989. For the same reason, the data reported in the HASBAP cannot directly be compared to studies conducted in other countries. One can be confident, however, that the control group design of the HASBAP ensures that comparisons *between* the four groups investigated can be interpreted in a meaningful way.

Table 4.8 shows the socio-economic status in the family of origin and patients' own social status at the time before the first episode of mental illness. Socio-economic status in the family of origin was determined through the occupation of the subject's father, or, if the occupation of the father was indeterminate, through that of the subject's mother. As can be seen, with regard to the socio-economic

Table 4.8. Socio-economic status (SES)

	ATPD $n = 42$	PS $n = 42$	BSAD $n = 42$	CNTR $n = 42$	
	n (%)	n (%)	n (%)	n (%)	Statistical analysis[a]
SES of family of origin					n.s.
Very high SES	1 (2.4)	2 (4.8)	0	2 (4.8)	
High SES	7 (16.7)	11 (26.2)	8 (19.0)	4 (9.5)	
Medium SES	9 (21.4)	5 (11.9)	7 (16.7)	6 (14.3)	
Low SES	20 (47.6)	17 (40.5)	22 (52.4)	28 (66.7)	
Very low SES	3 (7.1)	4 (9.5)	3 (7.1)	1 (2.4)	
Unclassifiable	2 (4.8)	3 (7.1)	2 (4.8)	1 (2.4)	
SES at onset of the disorder					ATPD > PS*
Very high SES	1 (2.4)	0	0		
High SES	6 (14.3)	1 (2.4)	2 (4.8)		
Medium SES	5 (11.9)	5 (11.9)	6 (14.3)		
Low SES	12 (28.6)	14 (33.3)	19 (45.2)		
Very low SES	3 (7.1)	6 (14.3)	3 (7.1)		
Unclassifiable	15 (37.5)	16 (38.1)	12 (28.6)		

SES, socio-economic status.

[a] Only pairwise comparisons with significant differences (Mann–Whitney U-test) are shown.

*$P < 0.05$, n.s. no significance.

status of the family of origin, no significant differences could be found between the clinical groups. Further, none of the clinical groups differed from the controls. In contrast, at the time before the onset of the disorder, a significant difference had emerged: patients with PS had a lower socio-economic status than those with ATPD. This finding is in concordance with the early social decline in schizophrenic patients found by the Cologne Study and many other investigations (Goldberg and Morrison, 1963; Wiersma *et al.*, 1983; Eaton, 1985; Angermeyer and Klusmann, 1987; Jones *et al.*, 1993), and indicates that this decline does not extend to ATPD.

Conclusion: Patients with Acute and Transient Psychotic Disorders have a higher socio-economic status than schizophrenic patients at the onset of the disorder, although there may be no differences in socio-economic status of the families of origin.

The further development of social status during the course of illness is discussed under 'Socio-economic status' on p. 154.

Table 4.9. Stable heterosexual relationship before onset

	ATPD $n = 42$	PS $n = 42$	BSAD $n = 42$	
	n (%)	n (%)	n (%)	Statistical analysis[a]
All patients				
Never	4 (9.5)	14 (33.3)	9 (21.4)	PS > ATPD**
Before, but not at onset	8 (19.0)	10 (23.8)	8 (19.0)	n.s.
Relationship at onset	30 (71.4)	18 (42.9)	25 (59.5)	ATPD > PS**
Only patients >25 years	$n = 36$	$n = 32$	$n = 20$	
Never	3 (8.3)	7 (21.9)	1 (5.0)	n.s.
Before, but not at onset	8 (22.2)	9 (29.0)	5 (25.0)	n.s.
Relationship at onset	25 (69.4)	16 (51.6)	14 (70.0)	n.s.

[a] Only pairwise comparisons with significant differences (χ^2 test or Fisher's exact test, two-tailed) are shown. **$P < 0.01$, n.s. no significance.

Stable heterosexual relationship before onset

Many studies have shown that in schizophrenia many patients do not have a stable heterosexual relationship even before the onset of the disorder (Schubart, 1986; Munk-Jørgensen, 1987; Marneros *et al.*, 1991b). Low premorbid rates of marriage and partnership differentiate patients with schizophrenia from patients with affective and schizoaffective disorders (Marneros *et al.*, 1991b).

In the study of Das and co-workers (1999) comparing 40 patients with ATPD and 40 patients with schizophrenia, more patients with schizophrenia were single at the onset of the illness than patients with ATPD, but the difference was not statistically significant.

In Table 4.9, the rates of stable heterosexual relationships in the clinical groups of the HASBAP up to the onset of the disorder are reported. A stable heterosexual relationship was defined operationally as one of at least six months duration. The main difference found concerns ATPD and PS: patients with PS significantly more often never had a stable heterosexual relationship before onset, and were significantly less often living in a stable heterosexual relationship at the onset of the disorder. Quite obviously, rates of partnership are influenced by the patients' age and gender. Very young people will have had less opportunity for long-term relationships than older people. The samples investigated in the HASBAP partially differ in age at onset (see p. 79). To compensate for these differences, the calculations were repeated after exclusion of all patients below the age of 25 at the onset of the disorder. In this subsample, the pattern of differences remained the same, but, mainly due to the smaller numbers, the differences were no longer significant.

Conclusion: More Acute and Transient Psychotic Disorder patients seem to have a stable heterosexual relationship than patients with Positive Schizophrenia until the onset of the disorder. In contrast, no difference between Acute and Transient Psychotic Disorders and Bipolar Schizoaffective Disorders can be observed in this regard. The differences between Acute and Transient Psychotic Disorders and schizophrenia are not statistically significant in small samples, but they are consistent across studies.

Traumatic experiences

Traumatic experiences in the history of patients with ATPD have only been investigated in the HASBAP. As traumatic experiences, events were defined which not only led to subjective distress, but which would normally be perceived as severely traumatic by most people. Examples include: being a victim of a violent crime, sexual abuse, surviving disaster or a life-threatening situation. In contrast to life events (see pp. 103ff), the traumatic experiences as defined above do not have to be temporally related to the onset of the episode.

A causal role of severe trauma for the later development of psychotic disorders is not generally accepted, although childhood sexual trauma seems to be associated with a broad range of psychopathological conditions (Wexler *et al.*, 1997; Bulik *et al.*, 2001; Simpson and Miller, 2002) and with poorer psychosocial functioning in adults with schizophrenia (Lysaker *et al.*, 2001). Some authors have reported psychotic symptoms in patients with posttraumatic stress disorder (Bleich and Moskowits, 2000; Ivezic *et al.*, 2000). In these cases, psychotic symptoms, such as delusions or auditory hallucinations, appeared months or even years after the psychological trauma (Bleich and Moskowits, 2000). The content of the psychotic experiences was related to the traumatic experience. The results of the HASBAP are given in Table 4.10. As can be seen, a large majority of the psychotic groups and almost all mentally healthy subjects did not report severe traumatic experiences during their lifetime. However, 16.6% of schizophrenic patients experienced traumatic experiences, mostly sexual abuse or rape, as did 12% of patients with ATPD and in almost 10% of BSAD. None of the mentally healthy people reported sexual abuse or robbery. The differences were significant only for PS patients in comparison with healthy controls. In none of the cases were the psychotic phenomena related to the trauma in content.

Table 4.10. Traumatic experiences

	ATPD $n = 42$	PS $n = 42$	BSAD $n = 42$	CNTR $n = 42$	
	n (%)	n (%)	n (%)	n (%)	Statistical analysis[a]
No traumatic experience	37 (88.1)	34 (81.0)	38 (90.5)	41 (97.6)	PS < CNTR*
Sexual abuse	2 (4.8)	4 (9.5)	2 (4.8)	0	n.s.
Rape	3 (7.1)	3 (7.1)	2 (4.8)	0	n.s.
Severe accident	0	0	0	1 (2.4)	n.s.
Other	0	1 (2.4)	0	0	n.s.

[a] Only pairwise comparisons with significant differences (χ^2 test or Fisher's exact test, two-tailed) are shown. *$P < 0.05$, n.s. no significance.

Conclusion: Lifetime traumatic experiences are uncommon in Acute and Transient Psychotic Disorders, Positive Schizophrenia and Bipolar Schizoaffective Disorder. There is no elevated rate of traumatic experiences in Acute and Transient Psychotic Disorders compared to Positive Schizophrenia and Bipolar Schizoaffective Disorders. But lifetime traumatic experiences are slightly more frequent in the clinical groups than in the healthy controls (significantly in schizophrenia).

Obstetric complications

Schizophrenia, particularly in its severe form, has been described as a 'neurodevelopmental disorder' (Murray, 1994; Marenco and Weinberger, 2000). According to this hypothesis, adult schizophrenia in general, or a subtype of schizophrenia, results from neurodevelopmental impairment early in life, including brain damage during the prenatal and perinatal period (Kunugi *et al.*, 2001). Evidence in favour of this hypothesis has been found in studies showing an increased risk of obstetric complications in new-borns diagnosed with schizophrenia later in life (McNeil *et al.*, 1994; Kunugi *et al.*, 2001).

It is unclear whether the reported increase of obstetric complications in schizophrenia extends to ATPD as well. On the one hand, proponents of the Leonhard classification of psychoses have postulated that cycloid psychoses show low heritability, but more exogenous disturbances during pregnancy and childbirth than patients with deteriorating 'systematic' schizophrenia (Stöber *et al.*, 1997). Following this line of reasoning, patients with ATPD would be expected to show *higher* rates of obstetric complications than schizophrenic patients. On the other hand,

Table 4.11. Obstetric complications

	ATPD $n = 42$	PS $n = 42$	BSAD $n = 42$	CNTR $n = 42$	
	n (%)	n (%)	n (%)	n (%)	Statistical analysis[a]
No complication reported	35 (83.3)	38 (90.5)	39 (92.9)	39 (92.9)	n.s.
Complications suspected	6 (14.3)	2 (4.8)	3 (7.1)	2 (4.8)	n.s.
Definite complications	1 (2.4)	2 (4.8)	0	1 (2.4)	n.s.

[a] No significant differences in pairwise comparisons with χ^2 test or Fisher's exact test.

obstetric complications in schizophrenia seem to be correlated with low premorbid functioning, a potent marker for subtypes of unfavourable prognosis (Kunugi *et al.*, 2001). From this point of view, ATPD patients would be expected to show *lower* rates of obstetric complications than patients with schizophrenia do.

Since no other study had investigated the issue, data on obstetric complications were collected only in the HASBAP. Obstetric complications were assessed through the subjects' own reports and information from sources and the hospital files of the patients. Obstetric files were not available for evaluation. Systematic and comprehensive interviews with the subjects' mothers were impracticable due to the high prevalence of 'broken home' situations (see p. 17) and the age structure of the sample. The completeness of the available information was therefore necessarily restricted. With this limitation considered the presence of obstetric complications was rated globally in three categories:

- no obstetric complications reported,
- complications suspected (e.g. prolonged labour),
- definite complications (e.g. asphyxia, low birth weight).

Table 4.11 shows the numbers of patients with a history of obstetric complications. As shown in Table 4.11, no significant differences emerged between ATPD, PS, BSAD and the mentally healthy controls.

> Conclusion: At present, the data do not support any notion of an excess of obstetric complications in patients with Acute and Transient Psychotic Disorder. This conclusion, however, is limited by the small number of patients investigated so far.

Early development

In schizophrenia, disturbances of early development, including abnormalities in motor behaviour, speech and social behaviours, have been documented extensively

Table 4.12. Disturbances of early development

	ATPD $n = 42$	PS $n = 42$	BSAD $n = 42$	CNTR $n = 42$	
	n (%)	n (%)	n (%)	n (%)	Statistical analysis[a]
No disturbance	40 (95.2)	37 (88.1)	36 (85.7)	42 (100)	PS < CNTR*
					BSAD < CNTR*
Suspected disturbance	1 (2.4)	3 (7.1)	5 (11.9)	0	n.s.
Definite disturbance	1 (2.4)	2 (4.8)	1 (2.4)	0	n.s.

[a] Only pairwise comparisons with significant differences (χ^2 test or Fisher's exact test, two-tailed) are shown. *$P < 0.05$, n.s. no significance.

(Nasrallah, 1993; Jones *et al.*, 1994; Asarnow, 1999). The most widely accepted explanation for this phenomenon is again the neurodevelopmental hypothesis of schizophrenia (Murray, 1994; Marenco and Weinberger, 2000) already discussed above. As with obstetric complications, no study had investigated the issue of early developmental abnormalities in ATPD until the HASBAP explored the subject.

In the HASBAP, abnormalities of early development were assessed primarily through the subjects' self-reports. The same sources of information, as was the case for obstetric complications, also applied to deviancies in early development. The assessment also had the same limitations. Disturbances of early development were defined as a disruption or delay of normal development before school age in one of the following domains: cognitive development, physical development (including motor behaviour, vision and hearing) and communication development including speech. They were also rated in three categories:

- no disturbances of early development,
- questionable disturbance of early development,
- definite disturbance of early development (documented delay in acquisition of language or delayed motor development).

Table 4.12 shows the numbers of patients with a history of developmental disturbance. Overall, there were few significant differences between the groups. It is noteworthy, however, that significantly more patients with PS and BSAD had disturbances of early development when compared with healthy controls, while there was no such difference between healthy control subjects and ATPD patients.

Conclusion: Early developmental abnormalities that have been implicated in the pathogenesis of schizophrenia might play a lesser or even no role in Acute and Transient Psychotic Disorders than in schizophrenia and schizoaffective disorder.

Premorbid personality and social interactions

While there is a large body of literature on the premorbid personality in schizophrenia and in affective disorders, much less is known on premorbid personality in schizoaffective disorders, and little on personality in ATPD (Marneros *et al.*, 1991b). In schizophrenic patients, the premorbid personality has most often been described as schizoid, adynamic, introverted and autonomically labile (Angst and Clayton, 1986; Marneros *et al.*, 1991b). With regard to affective disorders, there is now fairly consistent evidence of an elevated prevalence of obsessoid traits and 'typus melancholicus' features in unipolar depression (Tellenbach, 1976; von Zerssen, 1976, 2001; Sakado *et al.*, 1997). The premorbid personality of schizoaffective patients is less well investigated and seems to be more variable (Marneros *et al.*, 1991b).

With regard to the concepts of Brief and Acute Psychoses, the opinions seem to be divided. While some authors assume the premorbid personality to be basically intact (Leonhard, 1957; Ey, 1954), there is also a strong tradition of authors who believe Brief and Acute Psychoses occur preferentially in individuals with a particular personality, most often described as emotionally labile, easily impressed and prone to disproportionate affective reactions (Strömgren, 1986; Ungvari and Mullen, 2000) (see also above, p. 29ff). Concepts based on the theory of degeneration, including Magnan's bouffée délirante, implied a predisposing abnormality of the personality. This 'fragile personality' (Pichot, 1986b) was assumed to be the consequence of 'degeneration' (Magnan, 1893; Magnan and Legrain, 1895; Bonhoeffer, 1907; Schröder, 1920, 1922, 1926; Binswanger, 1928). Later, the proponents of emotional psychoses emphasised the interaction of emotional distress with an effectively labile personality (Staehelin, 1946; Störring *et al.*, 1962; Labhardt, 1963; Störring, 1969; Boeters, 1971). Although the concept of reactive psychosis focuses on psychosocial triggers, in many cases, a particular vulnerability of the personality is assumed (Strömgren, 1986).

However, despite the theoretical importance of the issue, little empirical data have been collected with relevance to the question of personality features in ATPD. An exception is the study of Jørgensen and co-workers (1996). The authors applied the International Personality Disorder Examination (IPDE) to their sample of 51 patients with ATPD after the patients were recovered. They found a relatively high prevalence (63%) of personality disorders. The spectrum of personality disorders according to ICD-10 was broad with five patients with anxious personality disorder, four patients with anankastic personality disorder, three patients with paranoid personality disorder, two patients with dependent personality disorder and one patient each with schizoid, emotionally unstable and histrionic personality disorder. By far the most frequent category, however, was unspecified personality disorder

($n = 15$). Thus, the authors could not observe a particular pattern in regard to the type of personality disorders. At the 1-year follow-up (Jørgensen *et al.*, 1997), the presence of personality disorders was reassessed. At that time, the prevalence of personality disorders had decreased to 46% (11 of 24 patients available for follow-up who were still believed to belong to the diagnostic category of ATPD). The distribution was not significantly changed. A limitation of the study of Jørgensen and co-workers (1996, 1997) is that the authors did not investigate a control group, and did not attempt to assess the premorbid state explicitly.

In the HASBAP, dimensional personality traits were assessed with the NEO-FFI, while the type of premorbid personality was rated by the clinical interviewer.

As a standardised and internationally recognised means of assessing the personality of patient groups and control subjects, the NEO five-factor inventory (Costa and McCrae, 1992) was administered. The self-rating scales were completed by the patients at the first follow-up point, outside the acute episode. Since the instrument was applied *after* the onset of illness, it assessed *postmorbid* personality features. It is unclear to what extent the self-rating at this point reflects premorbid features. However, temporal stability of the NEO five-factor inventory has been demonstrated in psychotic patients (Kentros *et al.*, 1997), as well as its good validation in psychiatric and non-psychiatric populations (Borkenau and Ostendorf, 1993; Blöink *et al.*, 2004). Results obtained with the NEO five-factor inventory in the HASBAP are given in Table 4.13. The assessment of personality features by applying the NEO-FFI after recovery from the acute episode showed that, in all subscales (neuroticism, extraversion, openness to experience, agreeableness, conscientiousness), the ATPD patients did not significantly differ from the mentally healthy group (Table 4.13).

Patients in the BSAD group differed from the mentally healthy control group in regard to neuroticism and extraversion, with higher scores for neuroticism and lower scores for extraversion in the BSAD patients (BSAS patients also showed lower scores for extraversion than ATPD patients). PS patients showed the same pattern of differences from the mentally healthy group, and had lower scores than the mentally healthy controls on the subscale 'conscientiousness'. The findings of the HASBAP are in agreement with the results of Gurrera and co-workers (2000), who found higher neuroticism and lower conscientiousness in patients with schizophrenia compared to controls from the community.

In the HASBAP, the assessment of 'premorbid' personality is subject to a number of limitations, many of which are common to most studies exploring premorbid personality in psychotic disorders. The most important limitation results from the fact that the patients were investigated *after* the manifestation of the illness. Additionally, some of the patients had several other psychotic episodes prior to the index episode. The information obtained from the patients themselves or from their relatives may, therefore, not always be reliable. The contamination of 'premorbid',

Table 4.13. Assessment of personality features with NEO-FFI

	ATPD $N = 35^a$	PS $n = 32^a$	BSAD $n = 37^a$	CNTR $n = 42$	
	Mean ± SD	Mean ± SD	Mean ± SD	Mean ± SD	Statistical analysis[b]
Neuroticism	1.89 ± 0.57	2.09 ± 0.60	2.10 ± 0.61	1.70 ± 0.55	$P = 0.009$ PS > CNTR[(*)] BSAD > CNTR*
Extraversion	2.11 ± 0.52	1.90 ± 0.53	1.76 ± 0.46	2.34 ± 0.49	$P < 0.001$ PS < CNTR** BSAD < CNTR*** BSAD < ATPD*
Openness for experiences	2.18 ± 0.37	2.00 ± 0.58	2.18 ± 0.49	2.24 ± 0.37	$P = 0.160$
Agreeableness	2.75 ± 0.41	2.70 ± 0.43	2.61 ± 0.52	2.52 ± 0.41	$P = 0.127$
Conscientiousness	2.76 ± 0.43	2.46 ± 0.68	2.53 ± 0.46	2.79 ± 0.43	$P = 0.012$ PS < CNTR[(*)]

[a] Patients unable to complete the questionnaire because of their symptoms excluded, therefore reduced n.
[b] P for ANOVA, only *post-hoc* comparisons significant in Scheffé procedure are indicated. * $P < 0.05$, ** $P < 0.01$, *** $P < 0.001$, [(*)] $P = 0.05$.

'morbid' and 'post-morbid' elements is difficult to avoid (Marneros *et al.*, 1991b, c). Features, which are already prodromal expressions of the disorder, especially in schizophrenia, could be erroneously taken as personality traits. The finer the personality details to be assessed, the more serious the danger of contamination. Despite these difficulties, a reliable assessment of premorbid personality features on a general level seems feasible, even in psychotic patients (Fritsch, 1975; Mundt, 1982, 1985; Sauer *et al.*, 1997).

In the HASBAP, it was attempted in every case to reconstruct the patients' premorbid personality from the participants' own reports, from the information given by family members and from the hospital files. Four typological categories were differentiated that have already been successfully applied to psychotic and affective patients in an earlier study (Marneros *et al.*, 1991b):

- Obsessoid: This personality type is characterised by orderliness, perfectionism, conscientiousness, industriousness and normal orientation.
- Asthenic/low self-confidence: This personality type is characterised by difficulties to develop initiative, difficulties with making decisions, hypersensitivity to criticism and rejection, feelings of inadequacy, insecurity in the pursuit of goals.

Table 4.14. Assessment of personality in the sociobiographic interview

	ATPD $n = 42$	PS $n = 42$	BSAD $n = 42$	
	n (%)	n (%)	n (%)	Statistical analysis[a]
Obsessoid	9 (21.4)	2 (4.8)	6 (14.3)	PS < ATPD *
Asthenic/low self-confidence	20 (47.6)	17 (40.5)	15 (35.7)	n.s.
Sthenic/High self-confidence	5 (11.9)	3 (7.1)	8 (19.0)	n.s.
Nervous-tense	4 (9.5)	7 (16.7)	4 (9.5)	n.s.
Undeterminable	4 (9.5)	13 (31.0)	9 (21.4)	ATPD < PS*

[a] Only pairwise comparisons with significant differences (χ^2 test or Fisher's exact test, two-tailed) are shown. *$P < 0.05$, n.s. no significance.

- Sthenic/high self-confidence: This personality type is largely the opposite of the asthenic/low self-confidence type: self-assured, active and easy in interpersonal relationships.
- Nervous-tense: This personality type is characterised by feelings of anxiousness, frequent worries, restlessness, and a tendency to be easily frightened.

If, after consideration of all sources of information, the patient could not be allocated to one of these categories, the premorbid personality was rated as 'undeterminable'. Because there was no way to define a 'premorbid' period in the mentally healthy controls, premorbid personality was only determined in the patient groups. Results of the assessment of premorbid personality are given in Table 4.14. Overall, little difference could be found between the three groups. As in the Cologne study (Marneros et al., 1991b), the highest rate of 'undeterminable' premorbid personality was found in the PS group (31.0%). In patients with schizophrenia it is particularly difficult to differentiate between early signs of the psychosis ('pre-episodic alterations') and preexisting personality features. The high rate of 'undeterminable' cases in the BSAP group may be related to the early onset of the disease in many of these patients which also makes the differentiation of premorbid personality difficult. The only significant difference found was a higher frequency of obsessoid personality features in ATPD patients than in PS patients. It is noteworthy that no elevated rates of the asthenic/low self-confidence or the nervous-tense type of personality were found in ATPD when compared to the other clinical groups. The findings of the HASBAP therefore do not support the assumption that ATPD preferentially occurs in emotionally labile personalities, as postulated by some authors (see p. 29ff). Rather, ATPD patients seem to be distinguished from PS by a higher frequency of

Table 4.15. Premorbid social contacts

	ATPD $n = 42$	PS $n = 42$	BSAD $n = 42$	
	n (%)	n (%)	n (%)	Statistical analysis[a]
Many social contacts	29 (69.0)	14 (33.3)	28 (66.7)	ATPD > PS**
				BSAD > PS**
Few social contacts	11 (26.2)	24 (57.1)	14 (33.3)	ATPD < PS**
				BSAD < PS*
Socially isolated	2 (4.8)	2 (4.8)	0	n.s.
Insufficient information		2 (4.8)		

[a] Only pairwise comparisons with significant differences (χ^2 test or Fisher's exact test, two-tailed) are shown. *$P < 0.05$, **$P < 0.01$, n.s. no significance.

obsessoid features (but only in a minority of patients), which have in many studies been associated with unipolar affective disorders (von Zerssen, 1976; Marneros et al., 1991c; Hecht et al., 1997; Mundt et al., 1997; Stanghellini and Mundt, 1997).

The quality of premorbid social interactions is linked closely to premorbid personality features (Marneros et al., 1991b). For schizophrenia in particular, a pattern of reduced social contacts and activities in the premorbid period has been described (Ellison et al., 1998). Therefore, the level of social interactions was recorded as an additional indicator of premorbid personality traits.

In the HASBAP, social interactions before the first episode of illness were recorded using information from the subjects' own reports, data from sources and data from case records. Social interactions were rated as 'many contacts' if subjects had a wide range of social contacts including several close relationships. Subjects were rated as 'few contacts' if they had only a limited number of social contacts including one close relationship outside the immediate family. Subjects were rated as socially isolated if they had no more than casual social contacts and no close relationship outside the immediate family before onset of the illness.

Results of this analysis are shown in Table 4.15. Two-thirds of patients in the ATPD group and BSAD group had 'many social contacts', whereas only one-third of the schizophrenic group had 'many social contacts'. In contrast, the majority of PS patients (57%) had 'few social contacts', but only 26% of the ATPD group and 33% of the BSAD group had 'few social contacts'. The difference between patients with Positive Schizophrenia and the other clinical groups was statistically significant.

Conclusion: The assessment of the 'Big Five' personality dimensions (neuroticism, extraversion, openness to experience, agreeableness, conscientiousness) with the NEO-FFI after the psychotic episode does not show any significant difference between Acute and Transient Psychotic Disorder patients and healthy controls. The NEO-FFI findings cannot differentiate between premorbid personality features and consequences of the illness. The absence of any significant differences between Acute and Transient Psychotic Disorder patients and mentally healthy controls, however, strongly suggests that postmorbid, and possibly also premorbid, personality of Acute and Transient Psychotic Disorder patients does not differ substantially from the general population. Bipolar Schizoaffective Disorder patients differ from mentally healthy controls on two of five subscales of the NEO-FFI (neuroticism and extraversion), but are otherwise indiscernible from Acute and Transient Psychotic Disorder patients and mentally healthy controls. In contrast, Positive Schizophrenia patients do not only show the most pronounced differences from the mentally healthy controls on the NEO-FFI (on three of five subscales: neuroticism, extraversion and conscientiousness), but also have significantly less premorbid social interaction than the clinical controls. While a contamination of premorbid and postmorbid aspects cannot be excluded, it seems certain that schizophrenic patients have the most pathological findings in terms of premorbid personality and premorbid social interactions (Marneros et al., 1991b; Dalkin et al., 1994; Cuesta et al., 1999; Kronmüller and Mundt, 1999). It also seems the distinctive premorbid features found in schizophrenic patients do not extend to Acute and Transient Psychotic Disorders. However, there are some similarities regarding premorbid personality and premorbid social interactions between patients with Acute and Transient Psychotic Disorder and schizoaffective patients.

5

The clinical features of the acute episode

Precipitating factors

The question of whether an increased rate of stressful events can be found preceding the onset of ATPD is of high theoretical interest. As was discussed on page 29ff, the concepts of 'reactive', 'psychogenic' and 'emotional' psychoses have influenced the formation of the category of 'ATPD'. According to these concepts, stressful events would be expected to play an important role in the pathogenesis of ATPD. There is no agreement, however, on this issue. Other concepts, including that of cycloid psychoses, do not postulate a special role for preceding stress. The authors of ICD-10 left the issue open – they did not include preceding stress as an obligatory diagnostic criterion (as DSM-III-R did in the category of Brief Reactive Psychosis), but they provided an option to code 'associated acute stress' as present or absent.

The ICD-10 specifier 'associated acute stress' must be regarded as 'narrowly defined' for two reasons. First, it requires a close temporal relationship (2 weeks) with the event and the onset of psychosis; and second, it requires that the event be particularly stressful in nature. In contrast, there is a long tradition of life-event research in psychotic and affective disorders which has shown that there may be elevated rates of a broad range of adverse events in a period of several months before the onset of a major affective episode or the onset of a psychotic episode (Paykel, 1990, 1994; Marneros, 1999; Mundt *et al.*, 2000).

Of the 51 ATPD patients of Jørgensen (1996), more than one-half (53%) experienced the first psychotic symptoms within 2 weeks of stressful events, typically estimated as mild or moderate psychosocial stressors ($n = 24$, 89%), and in only three patients (11%) was a severe stressor obvious.

In the study of Das and co-workers (1999) significantly more ATPD patients (13 of 40) experienced acute stress within 2 weeks prior to the onset of psychosis than patients with schizophrenia (3 of 40). The difference was statistically significant. The authors investigated the occurrence of stressful life events in patients with ATPD further, differentiating (1) different kinds of life events, (2) ATPD patients with and without a history of psychiatric disorders in first-degree relatives and (3) investigating life events occurring during a larger period of time up to 1 year prior to the onset of psychosis (Das *et al.*, 2001). They used the Presumptive Stressful Life Events Scale (PSLES), a 51-item checklist developed in the North Indian population and applicable even with illiterate and semi-literate people. This instrument probes a large number of different types of life event with accompanying stress scores for each event. For analysis, events were classified as desirable, undesirable and ambiguous and an overall stress score was calculated. When ATPD patients with and without a positive family history for psychiatric illness in first-degree relatives were compared, it turned out that 11 of the 13 patients with a stressful life event within 2 weeks prior to onset of psychosis had a positive family history. The life events included threat to life or death of a close family member in three patients each, and financial loss, threat of school failure and accident of family members in one patient each. When compared on the key variables of number of life events and stress scores as measured with the PSLES, the patients with a positive family history reported significantly fewer total number of life events as well as significantly lower stress scores than the patients without a family history of psychiatric illness. The numbers of subtypes of life events (desirable, undesirable and ambiguous) were not significantly different between the groups. In conclusion, ATPD patients with a positive family history of psychiatric disorder in their first-degree relatives reported significantly less stress prior to the onset of their acute psychotic illness than ATPD patients with a negative family history. The authors interpret this finding as support for the stress-vulnerability hypothesis in the aetiology of ATPD.

In the study of Sajith and co-workers (2002) stress within 2 weeks prior to the onset of psychosis was present in 31 of 45 patients with Acute Polymorphic Psychotic Disorder. In this study, the presence of a preceding psychosocial stressor was rated according to the DSM-III-R axis IV (APA, 1987). The presence of a life event, however, was not predictive of diagnostic stability after 3 years.

The HASBAP investigated whether there were differences in the rates of stressful events in the weeks and months prior to the onset of the acute episodes of ATPD and the clinical control groups. To comply with the ICD-10 criteria, and, at the same time, to allow for a comparison with the broader literature on stressful life events, two definitions were considered: a narrow definition strictly following ICD-10, and a broader definition which is in accordance with the criteria generally used in life-event research (Paykel, 1990).

For a coding of associated acute stress, ICD-10 requires the first psychotic symptoms to occur within about 2 weeks of one or more events that would be regarded as stressful to most people in similar circumstances, within the culture of the person concerned. Typical events would be bereavement, unexpected loss of partner or job, marriage, the psychological trauma of combat, terrorism or torture. According

Table 5.1. Acute stress within 2 weeks before the acute episode (narrow definition of ICD-10)

	ATPD $n = 42$	PS $n = 42$	BSAD $n = 42$
	n (%)	n (%)	n (%)
Acute stress	4 (9.5)	0	0
No acute stress	38 (90.5)	42 (100)	42 (100)

No significant differences in pairwise χ^2 tests.

Table 5.2. Number of stressful life events during the 6 months before the acute episode

	ATPD $n = 42$	PS $n = 42$	BSAD $n = 42$	
	n (%)	n (%)	n (%)	Statistical analysis[a]
No life event	24 (57.1)	33 (78.6)	32 (76.2)	ATPD < PS*
One	15 (35.7)	8 (19.0)	9 (21.4)	n.s.
Two	3 (7.1)	0	1 (2.4)	n.s.
Three	0	1 (2.4)	0	n.s.

[a] Only pairwise comparisons with significant differences (χ^2 test or Fisher's exact test, two-tailed) are shown. *$P < 0.05$, n.s. no significance.

to the Clinical Guidelines of ICD-10 (WHO, 1992), long-standing difficulties or problems should not be included as a source of stress in this context.

In the HASBAP, these criteria were not only applied to the ATPD patients, but also to the controls with PS and BSAD. The results are given in Table 5.1. It is clear that, in the sample of the HASBAP, acute stress precipitating the acute episode was only found in ATPD, although only in a very low frequency.

The presence of one or more stressful life events was also considered. A stressful life event was defined as any objective stressful change in circumstances (e.g. separation from spouse, becoming unemployed) that occurred up to 6 months before the onset of the episode and that was rated at least moderately distressful by the patient. The results of this analysis are reported in Table 5.2. The majority of all three psychotic groups did not have any precipitant, but 42.9% of the ATPD patients, 21.4% of the PS patients and 23.8% of the BSAD patients had at least one stressful life event before the onset of the acute episode. The difference between

Table 5.3. Types of stressful life events during the 6 months before the acute episode

	ATPD $n = 21^a$	PS $n = 11^a$	BSAD $n = 11^a$
	n	n	n
Death of significant other	5	1	0
Separation/divorce	2	2	1
Serious illness/operation	1	0	1
Change of job or school	1	1	1
Unemployment	2	0	3
Moving house	1	0	0
Serious problems in family	1	2	2
Serious problems at work	3	1	1
Serious financial problems	1	1	0
Major journey	1	0	2
Other	3	3	0

^{a} Numbers in this table refer to life events, not patients.
No significant differences between diagnostic groups (Fisher's exact test, two-tailed).

ATPD and PS was statistically significant. Table 5.3 gives the types of stressful life events involved. No particular pattern of life events emerged that could be thought to differentiate between the three clinical groups.

Conclusion: The ICD-10 specifier 'associated acute stress' is useless as defined in ICD-10. It seems to be a rare phenomenon in Acute and Transient Psychotic Disorder. Its specifying power for Acute and Transient Psychotic Disorders should be re-considered. However, the importance of precipitating factors in Acute and Transient Psychotic Disorders depends on the criteria used. It may be more useful to extend the time period for the coding of acute stress to life events during a longer period and to include mildly or moderately stressful events. Such events more often precede Acute and Transient Psychotic Disorders than schizophrenic episodes. But even then, a stressful life event is not characteristic for the majority of Acute and Transient Psychotic Disorders. Most importantly: The presence of a preceding life event seems to carry no prognostic significance in Acute and Transient Psychotic Disorder.

Acuteness of onset

Acute onset is one of the defining features of 'Acute and Transient Psychotic Disorders' according to the WHO. In the Diagnostic Criteria, acute onset is defined

Table 5.4. Mode of onset of the acute episode

	ATPD $n = 42$	PS $n = 42$	BSAD $n = 42$	
	n (%)	n (%)	n (%)	Statistical analysis[a]
Abrupt (<48 h)	18 (42.9)	5 (11.9)	4 (9.5)	ATPD > PS**
				ATPD > BSAD***
Acute (≤14 days)	24 (57.1)	15 (35.7)	19 (45.2)	ATPD > PS*
Subacute (>14 days)	n.a.	22 (52.4)	19 (45.2)	n.s.

[a] Only pairwise comparisons with significant differences (χ^2 test or Fisher's exact test, two-tailed) are shown. *$P < 0.05$, **$P < 0.01$, ***$P < 0.001$, n.s. no significance, n.a. not applicable.

as a crescendo development of a clearly abnormal clinical picture in about 2 weeks or less: 'There is an acute onset of delusions, hallucinations, incomprehensible or incoherent speech or any combination of these. The time interval between first appearance of any psychotic symptoms and the presentation of the fully developed disorder should not exceed 2 weeks' (WHO, 1993).

The WHO recommended that, for research purposes, the onset be further specified as either abrupt (onset within 48 hours) or acute (onset within more than 48 hours, but less than 2 weeks). This distinction between abrupt and acute onset is motivated by the assumption that patients with abrupt onset of psychotic symptomatology could have a better prognosis (see also p. 8).

It must be noted that the WHO definitions of onset do *not* imply that *any* sign of illness must be absent until 14 days or 48 hours before the full development of the disorder. Rather, the definitions of 'acute' and 'abrupt' refer to the 'change from a state without psychotic features to a clearly abnormal psychotic state'. The presence of unspecific prodromal symptoms of more than 2 weeks duration, including anxiety, depression, social withdrawal or mildly abnormal behaviour, are not precluded (see p. 8).

An abrupt onset (within 48 hours) has been noted in 21 of 51 (42%) ATPD patients by Jørgensen and co-workers (1996) and in 30 of 45 patients (66.7%) with Acute Polymorphic Psychotic Disorder by Sajith and co-workers (2002).

For the HASBAP, Table 5.4 gives the mode of onset following the ICD-10 definition, which has also been applied to PS and BSAD episodes. This table shows that an abrupt onset was quite frequent in ATPD (42.9%). An acute or abrupt onset (which is, by definition, present in 100% of the ATPD patients) was also found in 47.6% of the PS patients and in 54.2% of the BSAD patients. Acute onset can, therefore, by no means be regarded as specific for ATPD. Even an abrupt onset, though much rarer in the control groups, was still found in 11.9% of PS patients and in 9.5% of the BSAD patients.

> Conclusion: Since acuteness of onset is one of the defining criteria of Acute and Transient Psychotic Disorders, the finding of a more acute onset in Acute and Transient Psychotic Disorders than in controls with Positive Schizophrenia and Bipolar Schizoaffective Disorder comes to no surprise. Two conclusions could nevertheless be drawn from the above data. Firstly, a very high number of Acute and Transient Psychotic Disorders patients not only have acute onset, but also fulfil the strict ICD-10 criterion of abrupt onset within 48 hours, which could not be expected from the definition of Acute and Transient Psychotic Disorders alone. Secondly, neither abrupt nor acute onset are specific for Acute and Transient Psychotic Disorders. A considerable number of patients with Positive Schizophrenia and Acute and Transient Psychotic Disorders have an acute onset, and both disorders, though more rarely, may also have an abrupt onset.

Prepsychotic alterations: the so-called prodromal states

Psychiatric diagnoses are still a psychopathological convention and a compromise it is not justified to separate definitively between 'premorbid', 'intramorbid' and 'postmorbid'. All three states are conceptualised as different manifestations of the same disorder, and there are no strict scientific criteria to separate the so-called 'prodromal' states from 'core states' of psychotic disorders. The criteria so far proposed to separate 'prodromal' from 'core' states remain arbitrary (Marneros *et al.*, 1991b; Cornblatt *et al.*, 2001; McGorry *et al.*, 2001). It might therefore be more correct to define the so-called 'prodromal' state as '*prepsychotic* state', in contrast to the psychotic period. 'Psychotic' in this context is defined by the occurrence of productive forms of psychotic symptoms, namely delusions and hallucinations. In this sense and with a critical attitude towards the term 'prodromal', the terms 'initial symptoms' or 'prepsychotic symptoms' will be used interchangeably.

Although the ICD-10 definition of ATPD explicitly allows for a non-psychotic prodrome, little empirical data are available on the frequency and nature of such prodromal symptoms. Sajith and co-workers (2002), in their sample of 45 patients with Acute Polymorphic Psychotic Disorder, reported as most frequent non-psychotic symptoms: reduced sleep (97.8%) and reduced appetite (95.6%).

Non-psychotic initial symptoms in the three diagnostic groups of the HASBAP are shown in Table 5.5. The most frequent initial symptoms in all three psychotic groups were sleep disturbances. Depressed mood and reduced drive were also frequent initial symptoms, showing no significant difference between the three groups. Approximately one third of patients with ATPD and PS had anxiety, which differed

Table 5.5. Initial symptoms during the days before the onset of psychotic symptoms[a]

	ATPD $n = 42$	PS $n = 42$	BSAD $n = 42$	
	n (%)	n (%)	n (%)	Statistical analysis[b]
Sleepless	20 (47.6)	22 (52.4)	23 (54.8)	n.s.
Depressed, without drive	14 (33.3)	10 (23.8)	15 (35.7)	n.s.
Anxious, suspicious	13 (31.0)	16 (38.1)	3 (7.1)	ATPD > BSAD**
				PS > BSAD***
Dysphoric, agitated	11 (26.2)	11 (26.2)	24 (57.1)	ATPD < BSAD**
				PS < BSAD**
Maniform	7 (16.7)	1 (2.4)	20 (47.6)	ATPD < BSAD**
				PS < BSAD***
Ruminations	5 (11.9)	4 (9.5)	0	n.s.
Social retreat	1 (2.4)	6 (14.3)	1 (2.4)	n.s.
Cognitive disturbances	0	3 (7.1)	0	n.s.

[a] Several symptoms in one patient possible.
[b] Only pairwise comparisons with significant differences (χ^2 test or Fisher's exact test, two-tailed) are shown. ** $P < 0.01$, *** $P < 0.001$, n.s. no significance.

significantly from the group of BSAD patients, where anxiety was rarely an initial symptom.

While, on the whole, initial symptomatology did not distinguish well between ATPD and PS, two items are of interest in which ATPD patients and PS patients differed. In ATPD, maniform symptoms were found significantly more often than in PS. In PS, cognitive disturbances were found more often than in ATPD, but they were infrequent and the difference to ATPD fell just short of statistical significance ($P = 0.055$).

The differences between BSAD and the other two psychotic groups were more salient. In particular, the mood items (anxious/suspicious, dysphoric/agitated, and maniform) distinguished BSAD patients in the prepsychotic phase significantly from both ATPD and PS patients, with dysphoric and maniform symptomatology being more frequent in BSAD patients and anxiousness/suspiciousness being more frequent in ATPD and PS patients (Table 5.5).

Since the index episodes of the BSAD patients were not homogenous, but could be divided into schizomanic, schizodepressive and mixed schizoaffective episodes, an additional subgroup comparison was performed with regard to the prepsychotic symptomatology.

Of the bipolar schizoaffective controls, the index episode was schizomanic in 17 patients (40.5%), schizodepressive in 10 patients (23.8%) and mixed schizoaffective

Table 5.6. BSAD: type of index episode and prepsychotic symptoms

	Schizomanic (F25.0, $n = 17$)	Schizodepressive (F25.1, $n = 10$)	Mixed schizoaffective (F25.2, $n = 12$)	Statistical analysis[a]
	n (%)	n (%)	n (%)	
Mode of onset				
Abrupt (<48 h)	3 (17.6)	0	1 (8.3)	n.s.
Acute (2–14 days)	7 (41.2)	6 (60.0)	5 (41.7)	n.s.
Subacute (>14 days)	7 (41.2)	4 (40.0)	6 (50.0)	n.s.
Initial symptoms				
Sleepless	7 (41.2)	8 (80.0)	7 (58.3)	
Depressed, without drive	3 (17.6)	7 (70.0)	5 (41.7)	Schizomanic <Schizodepressive*
Anxious, suspicious	1 (5.9)	0	2 (16.7)	n.s.
Dysphoric, agitated	10 (58.8)	4 (40.0)	7 (58.3)	n.s.
Maniform	12 (70.6)	2 (20.0)	5 (41.7)	Schizodepressive <Schizomanic*
Ruminations	0	0	0	n.s.
Social retreat	0	0	1 (8.3)	n.s.
Cognitive disturbances	0	0	0	n.s.

[a] Only pairwise comparisons with significant differences (χ^2 test or Fisher's exact test, two-tailed) are shown.
*$P < 0.05$, n.s. no significance.

in 12 patients (28.6%). Three patients could not be classified (mainly schizodominant). Table 5.6 gives the acuity of the index episode and types of initial symptoms for the different subgroups of BSAD.

The only differences that emerged refer to the items 'depressed/without drive' and 'maniform', which are associated with the BSAD subtypes in the expected way.

> Conclusion: The prepsychotic alterations and initial symptomatology of Acute and Transient Psychotic Disorders are not specific. They are quite similar to that of Positive Schizophrenia, but shows more maniform and somewhat less cognitive symptoms. Some initial symptoms of Bipolar Schizoaffective Disorders, such as dysphoria, agitation and elation of mood are significantly more common in Bipolar Schizoaffective Disorders than in both Acute and Transient Psychotic Disorders and Positive Schizophrenia.

Table 5.7. Time course of the acute episode

	ATPD	PS	BSAD	
	$n = 42$	$n = 42$	$n = 42$	Statistical analysis[a]
Time from first psychotic symptom to full symptomatic picture in days				
Mean	3.9	41.1	27.5	$P < 0.001$
SD	3.9	55.7	45.1	ATPD < PS***
Median	3.0	15.5	14.0	ATPD < BSAD*
Range	0–14	0–221	0–271	
Time from first psychotic symptom to admission in days				
Mean	5.0	44.5	22.1	$P < 0.001$
SD	5.3	57.0	24.9	ATPD < PS***
Median	3.0	17.0	14.0	ATPD < BSAD*
Range	−3–20[b]	−21–221[b]	−14–271[b]	
Duration of psychotic period in days				
Mean	17.5	103.0	73.4	$P < 0.001$
SD	13.3	71.7	60.1	ATPD < PS***
Median	12.5	82.5	54.0	ATPD < BSAD***
Range	1–61	32–302	17–308	BSAD < PS*
Duration of inpatient treatment in days				
Mean	33.7	78.7	83.2	$P < 0.001$
SD	24.0	51.5	51.1	ATPD < PS***
Median	27.0	70.5	72.5	ATPD < BSAD***
Range	5–94	7–241	19–221	

[a] ANOVA: pairwise comparisons with significant differences (Scheffé procedure) are indicated.
*$P < 0.05$, *** $P < 0.001$.

[b] Negative values indicate onset of psychotic symptoms after admission.

The duration of the acute episode and its determinants

The duration of the psychotic episode is an important element of any operational definition of Brief and Acute Psychoses. But there is no consensus on the optimal duration criterion. As discussed above, Mojtabai, Susser and colleagues (2000) have argued that many Acute Brief Psychoses may have more than one, and even more than 2 month duration. They have suggested extending the possible duration of NARP to 6 months. In this case, however, overlap with the present criteria for schizophrenia would occur. For the patients of the HASBAP, detailed data were available on the time course of the acute episode. Table 5.7 gives a more complete overview of the time parameters and temporal evolution of the acute episode. Significant differences were found among the three groups of psychoses regarding the time that elapsed between the manifestation of the first psychotic symptom and the occurrence of the full symptomatology as defined in ICD-10. The interval for ATPD was 3.9 days, significantly shorter than for BSAD (27.5 days) or for PS (41.1 days).

The duration of the psychotic symptoms in ATPD, lasting 17.5 days, was significantly shorter than in schizoaffective disorder patients (73.4 days), which in turn was also significantly shorter than in schizophrenic patients (103.0 days). It is interesting that, in some patients with ATPD, a duration of the psychotic symptomatology of only 1 day was observed. The patients in all three groups received similar antipsychotic treatment. The duration of the inpatient treatment was significantly shorter in ATPD (33.7 days) than in PS (78.7 days) and BSAD (83.2 days).

The time from manifestation of the first psychotic symptoms to admission into the hospital was significantly shorter in ATPD than in PS. The difference between ATPD and BSAD, however, was not statistically significant. In some patients, in all three psychotic groups, the psychotic symptomatology (e.g. hallucinations, delusions) began after admission to the hospital (admission was necessary because of other nonpsychotic symptoms, such as disturbances of mood or of behaviour). This explains the 'minus' values in Table 5.7.

An interesting question is whether there is an interrelationship between the mode of onset of the acute episode, the presence of precipitating life events and the duration of the psychotic period.

The interrelationship of associated acute stress with the mode of onset was investigated by Jørgensen and co-workers (1996). In the majority of patients with associated stress ($n = 16$; 59%), the psychotic symptoms had an abrupt onset (occurring within 48 hours), whereas in patients without associated acute stress, an abrupt onset was less frequent ($n = 5$; 21%).

The findings of the HASBAP showed that, in the ATPD group, patients with or without precipitating life events during the 6 months before the acute episode did not differ significantly in the mode of onset, although there was a tendency for a more abrupt onset in patients with precipitating life events. The duration of the psychotic period was identical in patients with and without a stressful life event (Table 5.8). When the calculations were repeated for PS and BSAD, both groups showed a tendency for a shorter duration of the psychotic period when a stressful life event was present. When *all three clinical groups were considered together*, patients with or without precipitating life events during the six months before the acute episode did not differ significantly in the mode of onset, although there was a tendency for a more acute onset in patients with precipitating life events. The duration of the psychotic period was significantly longer in patients with a stressful life event than in patients without a life event (Table 5.9). In addition, a highly significant relationship was found between the mode of onset and the duration of

Table 5.8. Mode of onset of the acute episode and duration of psychotic period in patients with and without stressful life events in the six months preceding the acute episode (only patients with ATPD, $n = 42$)

	Without stressful life event $n = 24$	With stressful life event $n = 18$	
	n (%)	n (%)	Statistical analysis
Mode of onset			
Abrupt (<48 h)	9 (37.5)	9 (50.0)	n.s.[a]
Acute (≤14 days)	15 (62.5)	9 (50.0)	
Duration of psychotic period in days			
Mean ± SD	18.0 ± 14.7	16.8 ± 11.5	n.s.[b]

[a] χ^2 test.
[b] T-test.
n.s., no significance

Table 5.9. Mode of onset of the acute episode and duration of psychotic period in patients with and without stressful life events in the 6 months preceding the acute episode (all clinical groups, $n = 126$)

	Without stressful life event $n = 89$	With stressful life event $n = 37$	
	n (%)	n (%)	Statistical analysis
Mode of onset			
Abrupt (<48 h)	16 (18.0)	11 (29.7)	
Acute (≤14 days)	42 (47.2)	16 (34.2)	n.s.[a]
Subacute (>14 days)	31 (34.8)	10 (27.0)	
Duration of psychotic period in days			
Mean ± SD	72.1 ± 69.3	46.5 ± 48.3	0.042[b]

[a] χ^2 test.
[b] T-test.
n.s., no significance

the psychotic period (Table 5.10). In ATPD, the duration of the psychotic period was shorter for abrupt onset (<48 h) and longer for acute onset (≤14 days). In Positive Schizophrenia and in Bipolar Schizoaffective Disorder, patients with abrupt or acute onset had a shorter duration of the psychotic period than those with a subacute

Table 5.10. Duration of psychotic period in days according to mode of onset of the acute episode[a]

	ATPD		PS		BSAD	
Mode of onset	n	Mean ± SD	n	Mean ± SD	n	Mean ± SD
Abrupt (<48 h)	18	10.1 ± 8.2	5	77.2 ± 55.1	4	76.8 ± 73.6
Acute (≤14 days)	24	23.0 ± 13.8	15	76.9 ± 52.5	19	43.6 ± 33.7
Subacute (>14 days)			22	126.5 ± 80.1	19	102.4 ± 66.0

[a] In two-factor ANOVA significant main effects of mode of onset ($P < 0.001$) and diagnostic group ($P < 0.001$), interaction not significant. In *post hoc* pairwise comparisons the difference between patients with abrupt or acute onset and those with a subacute onset was highly significant, while the difference between patients with abrupt onset and those with acute onset was not significant.

onset. Statistical analysis confirmed a significant impact of the mode of onset on the duration of the psychotic period independent of diagnostic group. *Post hoc* analyses showed that the difference between patients with abrupt or acute onset and those with a subacute onset was highly significant in the Scheffé test, while the difference between patients with abrupt onset and those with acute onset was not significant.

> Conclusion: The duration of the psychotic period, as well as the duration of inpatient treatment, is significantly shorter in Acute and Transient Psychotic Disorders than in Positive Schizophrenia and Bipolar Schizoaffective Disorders. There is a significant tendency for patients with a more insidious onset to show a longer duration of the psychotic period. Additionally, there is a tendency for patients with a precipitating life event to show a more acute onset of the acute episode. These relationships hold true across diagnostic groups.

The symptoms of the acute episode

Already the early predecessors of ATPD such as 'cycloid psychoses' and 'bouffée délirante' have been thought to present with a more or less characteristic psychopathological picture. Most often this picture has been described as polymorphic, rapidly changing, or unstable.

The 'bouffées délirantes', as they were described at the end of the 19th Century in France by Valentin Magnan and Maurice Legrain, are psychotic disorders with acute onset and rapid remission characterised as 'délire d'emblée' (sudden madness) or 'bouffées subites d'idées délirantes' (Legrain, 1886). Regarded as typical were a sudden onset of delusional ideas and the rapid evolution of an intense symptomatology conferring different and often changing contents; they included megalomania, persecution and hypochondriasis. Pichot (1986a) described the delusional themes as numerous, diverse and protean (see p. 26). The delusions are a loose, motley jumble, without recognisable structure and cohesiveness. They may be accompanied by hallucinations. Eventually some degree of confusion exists with affective symptoms of various types ranging from anxiety, agitation, impulsiveness, and expansiveness to inertia.

Karl Kleist's conception of the 'cycloid psychoses' in their final delineation by Karl Leonhard with the three pairs of anxiety–happiness psychosis, excited–inhibited confusion psychosis and hyperkinetic–akinetic motility psychosis is mainly based on characteristic symptoms described in great detail in Leonhard's textbook (Leonhard, 1957, 1999). Common to all three types of cycloid psychoses is a bipolar structure with the ever-present possibility to switch from one pole to the other (see p. 18ff).

Thus, 'anxiety–happiness psychosis' is characterised by continuous changing between severe all-pervasive anxiety and ecstatic happiness. Anxiety is often associated with delusions and hallucinations. The experience of anxiety is overwhelming, but its intensity fluctuates, and the patients can suddenly turn to a state of ecstatic happiness. In the happiness–ecstasy phase the patients experience a feeling of revelation and of closeness to God. They feel like wanting to help others, to save them, to make them as happy as they themselves are. A peculiarity of the affects of this condition is their changing character during the episode. Clear-cut depressive or clear-cut manic mood is not recognisable or not long-lasting (Leonhard, 1961).

The 'excited-inhibited confusion psychosis' is characterised by thought disturbances, which in the excited type becomes incoherent accompanied by perplexity, whereas in the inhibited pole, does not proceed. Incoherence is mostly manifest in an inconsistent choice of themes or by an inconsistent use of different languages. In the most extremely inhibited form, the patient becomes mute. A wondering perplexity is present. Hallucinations and delusions are frequently present. Most often a polymorphous, rapidly changing pattern characterises the episodes of illness (Leonhard, 1961).

The main characteristic of the 'hyperkinetic–akinetic motility psychosis' is a disturbance of motility. In the hyperkinetic type, there is an increase in reactive and expressive movements and in pseudo-spontaneous movements. In contrast to the increased activity of many patients, they do not suffer pressure of speech. The patients remain mute in the hyperkinetic phase. In the akinetic phase, only a few isolated movements are carried out. In extreme cases, the patient may lie completely motionless in stupor and in cataplexia. The difference to catatonia lies in the fact that the way in which movements are carried out is not qualitatively disordered in motility psychoses (Leonhard, 1961).

It has to be noted, however, that later investigators did not always maintain Leonhard's sharp distinction of the three subtypes of cycloid psychoses (Cutting *et al.*, 1978; Brockington *et al.*, 1982b; Maj, 1988; Jönsson *et al.*, 1991b). Perris reported that, at the beginning of his landmark study of cycloid psychoses (Perris, 1974), it became evident that a clear-cut distinction among the three different subtypes of cycloid psychoses proposed by Leonhard was not always feasible (Perris, 1986). Although a few patients could be identified as belonging to one or other of the subtypes by the most dominant symptomatology in several episodes, an admixture of symptomatology appeared to be more the rule than the exception (Perris, 1986).

Jönsson conducted a number of factor analytic investigations using a historical cohort of inpatients admitted in 1925 to the hospital in Lund, Sweden. He tried to identify symptoms that discriminated cycloid psychoses from other psychotic disorders and predicted a remitting course (Jönsson *et al.*, 1991a,b; Jönsson, 1995). He found confusion, clouding of consciousness, happiness/ecstasy, anxiety/panic, global altruism and delusional mood.

In contrast to the historical descriptions, neither the criteria for ATPD nor those of BP require the presence of any particular symptom; just of psychotic symptoms in general. The investigation of unselected operationally diagnosed samples of ATPD and BP, therefore, provides an opportunity to validate the historical assumptions about the symptomatology of Brief and Acute Psychoses.

Sajith and co-workers (2002), in their sample of 45 patients with Acute Polymorphic Psychotic Disorder, reported as the most frequent psychotic symptoms: other auditory hallucinations (other than commenting voices or voices speaking in the third person) and delusions of persecution (91.1% and 82.2%, respectively).

In the HASBAP, the comparison of ATPD with the clinical control groups yielded a number of differences regarding symptomatology that merit discussion (Table 5.11). Delusions were generally equally frequent in all groups, but delusions of being influenced (including experiences of passivity) were found to be more frequent in schizophrenia. In contrast, the delusions of the ATPD group in comparison to the other two groups showed significantly more often a turbulent, changeable and dramatic character with rapidly changing topics. The frequency of hallucinations was significantly higher in the group of schizophrenic patients than in the other two groups. Surprisingly, the schizophrenic first-rank symptoms were represented almost equally at a high level in all three psychotic groups.

One of the most frequent symptoms in ATPD was anxiety, which was significantly more frequent than in schizophrenia or in Bipolar Schizoaffective Disorders. This finding is compatible with the concordance between Acute Polymorphic Psychotic Disorder and cycloid psychoses, especially the 'anxiety-elation psychosis' of the Wernicke–Kleist–Leonhard school (Pillmann *et al.*, 2001; Pillmann and Marneros, 2003). More than two-thirds of patients with ATPD experienced quickly changing

Table 5.11. Symptomatology of the acute episode

	ATPD $n = 42$	PS $n = 42$	BSAD $n = 42$	
	n (%)	n (%)	n (%)	Statistical analysis[a]
Productive psychotic symptoms (hallucinations or delusions)	42 (100)	42 (100)	42 (100)	n.s.
Hallucinations	32 (76.2)	39 (92.9)	32 (76.2)	PS > ATPD* PS > BSAD*
Delusions	41 (97.6)	41 (97.6)	38 (90.5)	n.s.
Delusions of being influenced	21 (50.0)	30 (71.4)	23 (54.8)	PS > ATPD*
First-rank symptoms	30 (71.4)	36 (85.7)	34 (81.0)	n.s.
Rapidly changing delusions	20 (47.6)	0	1 (2.4)	ATPD > PS*** ATPD > BSAD***
Affective disturbance	42 (100)	41 (97.6)	42 (100)	n.s.
Disturbance of drive and psychomotor disturbances	36 (85.7)	39 (92.9)	41 (97.6)	n.s.
Depressed mood	31 (73.8)	37 (88.1)	30 (71.4)	n.s.
Maniform symptoms	32 (76.2)	24 (57.1)	36 (85.7)	BSAD > PS**
Anxiety	32 (76.2)	22 (52.4)	22 (52.4)	ATPD > PS* ATPD > BSAD*
Rapidly changing mood	29 (69.0)	1 (2.4)	5 (11.9)	ATPD > PS*** ATPD > BSAD***
Thought disorder	36 (85.7)	41 (97.6)	41 (97.6)	n.s.
Bipolar character of symptoms	12 (28.6)	1 (2.4)	9 (21.4)	ATPD > PS*** BSAD > PS**

[a] Only pairwise comparisons with significant differences (χ^2 test or Fisher's exact test, two-tailed) are shown. *$P < 0.05$, **$P < 0.01$, ***$P < 0.001$, n.s. no significance.

moods. In almost 29% of the patients, the changes of mood had a bipolar form with an alternation between a depressive and a maniform pole. Although also in Bipolar Schizoaffective Disorders, 21% of patients alternated during the episode between depression and manic symptomatology and vice versa ('mixed states'). The changes in ATPD were more dramatic, more unstable and of shorter duration than in bipolar schizoaffective mixed states.

The symptomatological features, in particular the quickly changing state of mood, confirmed the relationship of ATPD to cycloid disorders (Leonhard, 1957, 1961, 1995, 1999; Perris, 1986; Marneros, 1999; Pillmann *et al.*, 2001) and to the bouffée délirante (Pichot, 1986; Pillmann and Marneros, 2003).

Special psychopathological aspects of ATPD

Both the various predecessors of ATPD the ATPD itself as defined by the WHO, have some characteristic psychopathological features which are described below.

An increased rate of patients with *visual hallucinations* has been noted by Cutting and co-workers (1978) and Maj and co-workers (1990a) for cycloid psychoses. The HASBAP found for ATPD that visual hallucinations occurred in ca. 17% of the patients and haptic or coenesthetic hallucinations in 14%. But *auditory hallucinations*, although somewhat less frequent in ATPD than in PS, are the most common. In ATPD, they most often occurred in the form of voices, in particular commanding voices (47.6%), commenting voices (35.7%) and voices in dialogue (23.8%). But the visual hallucinations are usually very vivid as the following case report shows:

During the psychiatric examination, the 45-year-old female patient with clear consciousness stared out of the window and reported that she saw her husband as a little mannequin dancing in a tree. Sometimes he had the light of life on his chest, sometimes it moved into his eye. A mask was also flying about in the tree showing a female and a male face in turn. Black and white birds in large numbers were also flying about in the tree.

Delusional topics in HASBAP patients were widespread and included delusions of reference (78.6%), delusions of persecution (61.9%), religious delusions (9.0%), delusions of guilt (14.3%), grandiose delusions ($n = 8$, 19.0%) and other topics. Delusional misidentification of individuals, which has been regarded as typical for ATPD, was quite frequent (38.1%).

One subject believed another patient on the ward to be her mother, one subject believed a passer-by to be her uncle who had died 2 years earlier, and another subject believed himself to be exchanged for another person he was acquainted to.

Religious topics were involved in more than a quarter of the sample (26.2%):

Patients started thinking about religious matters, went to a religious service where they interrupted the sermon, felt directed by God, or wanted to sacrifice themselves for God.

A *preoccupation with thoughts about death* (other than suicidal ideas) was experienced by two subjects:

One patient was convinced that she had killed her husband (who was present during the examination). Another patient experienced a growing fear of death, which at one point, when he was climbing up a staircase, became more and more intense. When he reached the last step, he was suddenly aware that everybody in the world was dead, and he himself was the only remaining living person.

Preoccupation with death has been described as typical for cycloid psychoses by Perris (1974).

Most often, patients worried about death or held the delusional belief that a close relative had died.

The *polymorphous symptomatology*, i.e. the main characteristic that distinguishes ATPD from the other two psychotic groups (PS and BSAD), was found in the form of rapidly changing delusional topics and other productive psychotic phenomena.

A 37-year-old physical therapist developed, literally over-night, a multitude of delusional and hallucinatory experiences in rapid succession: within a few hours she believed herself to be pregnant, a certain book contained special references to her, she felt persecuted by construction workers, and she experienced optical, auditory and coenaesthetic hallucinations accompanied by disturbances of speech, affect and motor behaviour.

Another example of polymorphic symptomatology in a patient with severe preceding stress was given by Jørgensen and co-workers (1996):

A 31-year-old woman realised within a few days that (1) she was pregnant and (2) she had malignant breast cancer. During the following 24 hours, her mental state changed in a turbulent way. She presented with an unstable, rapidly changing clinical picture including emotional turmoil, disordered perception, disorganised speech, transient hallucinations and delusions (Jørgensen et al., 1996).

A *bipolarity of mood* was found in 28.6% of ATPD subjects of the HASBAP, and in the most typical instances, manifested itself in the form of a co-existence of ecstatic feelings and feelings of anxiety, often accompanied by accordingly tainted productive symptoms:

A 24-year-old cook experienced the onset of her psychotic episode immediately after a dental treatment. She described an ecstatic feeling of happiness combined with the anxiety that something dreadful would happen. The bipolar nature of the affect was mirrored by the contents of her delusions and hallucinations: she was at one time convinced to be a princess of high birth, and shortly afterwards she was troubled by voices accusing her of having abused her son.

Conclusion: The most crucial differences regarding phenomenology among Acute and Transient Psychotic Disorders, schizophrenic and schizoaffective patients are 'rapidly changing delusional topics', 'rapidly changing mood' and 'anxiety'. All three are significantly more frequently represented in Acute and Transient Psychotic Disorders and are responsible for their highly dramatic picture. A bipolarity of mood (changes from depressive syndrome to excitation) is almost equally represented in Acute and Transient Psychotic Disorders and Bipolar Schizoaffective Disorders (due to 'mixed states'), but is almost unknown in schizophrenia (see Table 5.11).

6

Treatment

There are few systematic data regarding treatment of the predecessors of ATPD. Treatment of the acute episode with electroconvulsive therapy has been advocated for 'atypical psychoses' (Kurosawa, 1961) and 'cycloid psychoses'. A rapid response of cycloid psychoses to ECT has been supported by Kirov (1972), Mattson and Perris (1973) and Perris (1974). Neuroleptic treatment has also been recommended (Neumann and Schulze, 1966). For the long-term prophylaxis of cycloid psychoses, lithium therapy has been described as effective (Mattsson and Perris, 1973; Perris and Smigan, 1984).

Data on medication at the end of the acute episode of ATPD are given by Jørgensen and co-workers (1996) in their study on 51 patients. At the time of assessment the patients were non-psychotic; nevertheless most of them ($n = 42$; 82%) were taking antipsychotics and other psychotropic drugs ($n = 27$; 53%). Five patients (10%) were drug-free at the time of the interview.

The HASBAP was naturalistic with regard to treatment. It was decided that the treatment of the patients would depend upon the symptomatology according to clinical guidelines, and not to a rigid standardised schedule. The reason for this decision was based on the fact that there is no standardised knowledge on the treatment of Acute and Transient Psychotic Disorders in the literature, in contrast to schizophrenia, and to some extent, also in comparison to Bipolar Schizoaffective Disorders, where treatment guidelines do exist. Another reason was the acute and dramatic symptomatology of many patients of the ATPD group, which usually demands flexible treatment strategies and usually does not allow systematic double blind and placebo controlled studies.

Table 6.1 reports the numbers and proportion of patients who were treated with particular classes of drugs. All patients (with the exception of two ATPD patients and one BSAD patient) received antipsychotics (Table 6.1). In the group of ATPD and PS, antidepressants were the second most frequently administered medications (in both groups 21.4%), while in the group of Bipolar Schizoaffective Disorders, this position was occupied by lithium (47.6%). But only three patients

Table 6.1. Treatment in the episode

	ATPD $n = 42$	PS $n = 42$	BSAD $n = 42$	
	n (%)	n (%)	n (%)	Statistical analysis[d]
Antipsychotics	40 (95.2)	42 (100)	41 (97.6)	n.s.
Antidepressants	9 (21.4)	9 (21.4)	16 (38.1)	n.s.
Lithium	3 (7.1)	1 (2.4)	20 (47.6)	BSAD > ATPD***
				BSAD > PS***
Carbamazepine	2 (4.8)	1 (2.4)	12 (28.6)	BSAD > ATPD**
				BSAD > PS***
Valproate	0	0	4 (9.5)	n.s.
Benzodiazepine	29 (69.0)	21 (50.0)	19 (45.2)	ATPD > BSAD*
Monotherapy (only one specific[a] medication)[b]	27 (64.3)	32 (76.2)	7 (16.7)	ATPD < BSAD***
				PS < BSAD***
No specific medication[c]	2 (4.8)	0	0	n.s.

[a] Specific medication = antipsychotics, antidepressants or mood stabiliser.
[b] In virtually all cases an antipsychotic; only in one BSAD patient an antidepressant.
[c] i.e. tranquillizer only.
[d] Only pairwise comparisons with significant differences (χ^2 test or Fisher's exact test, two-tailed) are shown.
*$P < 0.05$, **$P < 0.01$, ***$P < 0.001$, n.s. no significance.

with ATPD, and only one patient with PS, received lithium during the acute episode. Approximately 29% of BSAD patients received carbamazepine, but only one patient with PS and two patients with ATPD received it. In other words, while 76% of BSAD patients received mood stabiliser, only 5% of patients with PS, and 12% of patients with ATPD received the same. Two-thirds of patients with ATPD, and one-half of patients with PS, and almost the same proportion in the group of BSAD, needed benzodiazepines during the episode; this is mainly true at the beginning because of agitation, or more usually, due to sleep disturbances. Benzodiazepines were only an adjuvant medication. Excluding the application of benzodiazepines, two-thirds of patients with ATPD had a monotherapy with only antipsychotics, not differing significantly from patients with PS. But only seven patients (16.7%) in the BSAD group received a monotherapy with antipsychotics. Most of them had a combination with a mood stabiliser.

For psychotic and major affective disorders, it is standard procedure to continue the psychopharmacological treatment beyond the point of discharge to prevent early relapse (APA, 1997; Marneros, 1999). In some cases, medication is continued in a long-term fashion as a prophylaxis against a recurrence of the disorder.

Table 6.2. Medication at discharge

	ATPD $n = 42$	PS $n = 42$	BSAD $n = 42$	
	n (%)	n (%)	n (%)	Statistical analysis[a]
No specific[b] medication at discharge	3 (7.1)	0	1 (2.4)	n.s.
Antipsychotic	38 (90.5)	42 (100)	37 (88.1)	n.s.
Antidepressant	8 (19.0)	7 (16.7)	16 (38.1)	PS < BSAD*
Lithium	3 (7.1)	0	15 (35.7)	ATPD < BSAD**
				PS < BSAD***
Carbamazepine	2 (4.8)	0	9 (21.4)	ATPD < BSAD*
				PS < BSAD***
Valproate	0	0	4 (9.5)	n.s.

[a] Only pairwise comparisons with significant differences (χ^2 test or Fisher's exact test, two-tailed) are shown. *$P < 0.05$, **$P < 0.01$, ***$P < 0.001$, n.s. no significance.

[b] Specific medication = antipsychotics, antidepressants or mood stabiliser.

Medication status at discharge, therefore, reflects the clinical judgement that a continued pharmacotherapy is necessary.

Table 6.2 shows that almost all patients in the three psychotic groups received medication at discharge. Only three patients in the ATPD group, and one patient with Bipolar Schizoaffective Disorder, were medication-free. A comparison with Table 6.2 shows that almost all patients continued antipsychotic medication initiated in the episode, with the exception of four patients in the ATPD group, one patient in the PS group, and five patients in the BSAD group. The proportion of patients receiving mood stabiliser remained almost unchanged in comparison to the medication during episode. The above data are entirely descriptive and naturalistic. It can be said, however, that in the overwhelming majority of cases, the clinical picture did not warrant stopping the medication already in use during the course of inpatient treatment. Continued pharmacotherapy was the rule, most often with antipsychotics, but in some cases also with lithium or other mood stabilisers as recommended by some authors for cycloid psychoses (Mattsson and Perris, 1973; Perris, 1978; Perris and Smigan, 1984). Recently, Dietrich and co-workers (2004) reported the successful treatment with Lamotrigine of four patients with 'confusion psychoses', a subgroup of cycloid psychoses according to Leonhard which had not responded to other mood stabilisers or antipsychotics. The proportion of patients treated with carbamazepine, valproate or the newly introduced mood stabilisers, will possibly increase in the future, as these substances appear to be helpful especially in atypical, mixed and 'rapid cycling' psychotic disorders (Calabrese et al., 2000).

Table 6.3. Treatment status at the end of the prospective follow-up period

	ATPD $n = 38$	PS $n = 34$	BSAD $n = 34$	
	n (%)	n (%)	n (%)	Statistical analysis[a]
Outpatient psychiatric treatment	28 (73.7)	31 (91.2)	33 (97.1)	ATPD < BSAD**
Psychotherapy	3 (7.9)	0	0	n.s.
Pharmacotherapy	27 (71.1)	30 (88.2)	33 (97.1)	ATPD < BSAD**
Antipsychotics	25 (65.8)	30 (88.2)	27 (79.4)	ATPD < PS*
Antidepressants	10 (26.3)	5 (14.7)	12 (35.3)	PS < BSAD*
Mood stabiliser	7 (18.4)	2 (5.9)	27 (79.4)	ATPD < BSAD***
				PS < BSAD***

[a] Only pairwise comparisons with significant differences (χ^2 test or Fisher's exact test, two-tailed) are shown. *$P < 0.05$, **$P < 0.01$, ***$P < 0.001$, n.s., no significance.

As we have seen in the HASBAP, nearly all of the patients in all three groups were on a psychotropic medication at the end of the acute episode when they were discharged from the hospital. It is of interest how many patients were still (or again) on medication at the time of follow-up, and how many patients were in psychiatric or psychotherapeutic treatment. The fact that a particular patient is receiving treatment at a certain point in time certainly does not directly imply the need for treatment, nor does the absence of treatment directly imply that treatment is no longer necessary. Indeed, the actual treatment status is also influenced by the demands of the patient and his or her compliance. Nevertheless, at least in the patients in the sample in the HASBAP who showed high compliance with the follow-up interviews, treatment rates seem to reflect, to a reasonable degree, the requirement for ongoing treatment.

In the study of Jørgensen and co-workers (1997), 10 of 24 (42%) patients with ATPD were taking psychotropic medication at the time of the 1-year follow-up, eight patients (33%) were taking antipsychotics and seven patients (29%) were taking antidepressants.

Table 6.3 reports the treatment status for all groups of the HASBAP at the end of the prospective follow-up period. Almost all patients with Bipolar Schizoaffective Disorders (with only one exception) and most patients with schizophrenia (with only three exceptions) received pharmacological or outpatient psychiatric treatment. In contrast, eleven patients with ATPD did not receive pharmacological treatment at the end of the prospective follow-up, and nine patients with ATPD did not receive any treatment at all. Further analysis showed that all of these patients had a GAS greater than 80 (most of them even greater than 90) indicating a very good general functioning. Patients without pharmacotherapy at the end of the prospective observation time also had fewer episodes during follow-up than patients with pharmacotherapy (mean number of episodes 0.91 vs. 1.96, difference significant in two-tailed t-test with $P = 0.03$). These analyses suggest that, in the majority of these patients, pharmacotherapy was not stopped because of non-compliance, but because of a favourable course.

With regard to the type of medication, the most frequently given drug in all three groups were antipsychotics while antidepressants were given in almost equal frequency in both Acute and Transient Psychotic Disorders and Bipolar Schizoaffective Disorders. The vast majority of patients with schizoaffective disorders also received a mood stabiliser (79%), as did 18% of the patients with ATPD. Only two patients in the schizophrenic group received a mood stabiliser. In essence, there was little change in the type of medication when compared to the medication at discharge (see page 69).

Conclusion: A small minority of patients with very short durations of psychotic symptoms remit before specific pharmacotherapy is started. The main medications in Acute and Transient Psychotic Disorders are antipsychotics. But Acute and Transient Psychotic Disorder patients also need tranquillisers, underscoring the dramatic clinical picture often accompanied by anxiety. Some patients with Acute and Transient Psychotic Disorders also need antidepressant therapy or a mood stabiliser, but the vast majority of patients can be treated with only one antipsychotic.

In a small group of Acute and Transient Psychotic Disorder patients, it appears to be possible to stop medication during long-term course. About two-thirds of Acute and Transient Psychotic Disorders patients in the Halle Study on Brief and Acute Psychoses patients could still be treated with antipsychotics at follow-up, which is significantly less than in patients with schizophrenia. Although a number of Acute and Transient Psychotic Disorder patients are receiving antidepressants or mood stabilisers, future research will have to show whether these treatments, in particular mood stabilisers, can substitute for treatment with antipsychotics in Acute and Transient Psychotic Disorders.

7

The longitudinal course

The typical course of Brief and Acute Psychoses has been described as remitting and relapsing. This is true for most historical predecessors of what we today call Acute and Transient Psychoses, especially for the cycloid psychoses which are believed to occur in recurring episodes, interrupted by symptom-free intervals. Leonhard (1957) found the duration of episodes in cycloid psychoses shorter than in manic-depressive illness and a lower number of episodes over the whole course of illness. The relatively short duration of cycloid episodes was confirmed by most later investigators (Kirov, 1972; Perris, 1974; Kimura *et al.*, 1980; Bräunig and Fimmers, 1995).

The duration of the cycle, i.e. the period of time comprising an illness episode and the ensuing interval, was reported by Perris (1974) with a mean of 2 years, but about twice that long between the first two episodes. This is similar to affective and schizoaffective disorders – both unipolar and bipolar (Angst *et al.*, 1980; Marneros *et al.*, 1989b, 1991b; Angst and Preisig, 1995). A further reduction of cycle length during long-term course as known for bipolar affective and schizoaffective psychoses was not identified by Perris in his data (1974). Kirov in his series of cycloid psychoses, found a free interval between two episodes of 20.3 months (Kirov, 1972). Of a similar order of magnitude are the findings of Cutting (1978), who found a relapse rate of 0.28 episodes/year, and those of Bräunig (1995), who reported an average of 3 episodes per year.

Perris (1974) calculated the number of episodes during the observation period separately for patients with homotypical heredity, heterotypical heredity and without heredity. The differences among groups were insignificant. Over a mean observation time of 12 years, about 5 episodes occurred.

Among the investigations of samples with ATPD defined according to ICD-10, Sajith and co-workers included only first-episode patients (2002), and Das and co-workers (1999, 2001) gave no information on earlier episodes, so that nothing can be said about real relapse patterns. Similarly, the sample of Jørgensen and co-workers (1996) included some patients with earlier episodes, but no information was given on these episodes except that the patients never previously fulfilled the diagnostic criteria of schizophrenia or affective disorder. Jørgensen and co-workers (1996) found that after 1 year, 15 of 46 patients (33%) available for follow-up had been readmitted because of a psychotic relapse. Non-psychotic relapses and non-readmitted relapses were not assessed.

In the study of Sajith and co-workers (2002), consecutive inpatients meeting ICD-10 research criteria for ATPD, polymorphic subtype without symptoms of schizophrenia (F23.0), were followed-up over a period of up to 3 years. Three-year follow-up data were available for 45 of the 52 patients. At that time, 24 of the patients had no further episodes, 8 had one further episode of ATPD, and 1 patient had two episodes of ATPD. Twelve patients had further episodes other than ATPD and underwent diagnostic change, mainly to bipolar disorder.

Two studies conducted on patients with 'Non-affective Acute Remitting Psychoses' (NARP) have reported relapse rates considerably lower than the numbers reported above (Susser et al., 1995a, 1998). However, they applied criteria differing from ICD-10 and DSM-IV, as well as from each other (as discussed on p. 44). In the Indian study of Susser and co-workers (1998), the criteria of Acute Brief Psychoses included freedom from relapse at the 2-year follow-up (otherwise a diagnosis of acute relapsing psychosis was assigned). Remarkably, only 18% of the patients relapsed within 12 years. Obviously, in this sample, freedom from relapse after 24 months (despite discontinuation of pharmacotherapy in most cases) strongly predicted freedom of relapse after 12 years. However, these results cannot be generalised to all cases of ATPD or BPLD, the definitions of which do not contain a criterion of relapse-free survival. In addition, prevalence differences between industrialised and developing countries could also contribute to the difference between the studies. Brief and Acute Psychoses appear to be more frequent in developing countries and may carry a better prognosis (Cooper and Sartorius, 1977; Jablensky et al., 1992; Susser et al., 1995b, 1998; Collins et al., 1996; Malhotra et al., 1998; Hopper and Wanderling, 2000).

The diagnostic criteria used in the North American study of Susser and co-workers (1995a) are more similar to ICD-10 criteria of ATPD, but they contain the requirement of a state of complete remission at (not within) 6 months after initial evaluation. This criterion might have excluded some patients with early relapse. In addition, the size of this sample was really very small ($n = 7$).

The most comprehensive assessment of episode frequency and episode types was performed in the German study. The findings of this study are reviewed on the following pages.

The HASBAP: types and frequencies of episodes

For a substantial number of patients, the episode at the beginning of the prospective follow-up was not the first episode of the disorder: 45.2% of the ATPD patients,

Table 7.1. Frequency of previous episodes until the beginning of the prospective follow-up

	ATPD $n = 42$	PS $n = 42$	BSAD $n = 42$	
	n (%)	n (%)	n (%)	Statistical analysis
No previous episode	23 (54.8)	16 (38.1)	2 (4.8)	ATPD > BSAD***[a] PS > BSAD***
At least one previous episode	19 (45.2)	26 (61.9)	40 (95.2)	
Number of previous episodes (mean ± SD)	1.6 ± 3.0	1.8 ± 2.0	5.2 ± 3.4	$P < 0.001$[b] ATPD < BSAD*** PS < BSAD***
Range	0–16	0–7	0–13	

[a] Only pairwise comparisons with significant differences (χ^2 test or Fisher's exact test, two-tailed) are shown. *** $P < 0.001$.

[b] ANOVA: pairwise comparisons with significant differences (Scheffé procedure) are indicated. *** $P < 0.001$.

61.9% of the PS patients, and even 95.2% of the BSAD patients, had earlier episodes. Table 7.1 gives details on the numbers of previous episodes for all groups. The most conspicuous finding is the high number of previous episodes in the BSAD sample. The differences to both ATPD and PS are highly significant. For the interpretation of these differences, it has to be kept in mind that in many cases of bipolar disorders, the initial course appears to be unipolar. One often has to wait for several episodes until the diagnosis of a bipolar disorder can be made (Goodwin and Jamison, 1990). This is certainly one reason for the higher number of previous episodes in BSAD, although the magnitude of the difference makes it unlikely the sole explanation. A second reason can be found in the very low age at onset that can be seen in many of the BSAD patients (see p. 79). An onset in early adulthood, or even adolescence, is not uncommon for bipolar disorders (Angst 1966, Marneros 1999).

Table 7.2 gives the types of previous episodes until the index episode, classified according to ICD-10 criteria (see p. 63). It has to be noted that, in some cases, the information on some of these episodes was limited. Although hospital records for every single episode of illness were obtained wherever possible, some of these episodes occurred decades ago, were treated abroad or were otherwise poorly documented. In some cases, after considering all available information, the diagnosis had to remain 'not classifiable' (see Table 7.2). Table 7.2 illustrates the fact that, in the selection of the index group with ATPD, patients who had experienced episodes other than ATPD at an earlier point in time were not excluded. Although earlier ATPD episodes were by far the most frequent ones in this group, 21.2% of the earlier

Table 7.2. Type of previous episodes until index episode

ICD-10 episodes	ATPD $n = 66^a$ n (%)	PS $n = 74^a$ n (%)	BSAD $n = 220^a$ n (%)	Statistical analysis[b]
ATPD	31 (47.0)	1 (1.4)	1 (0.5)	ATPD > PS*** ATPD > BSAD***
Depressive episode	14 (21.2)	0	40 (18.2)	ATPD > PS*** BSAD > PS***
Manic episode	2 (3.0)	0	24 (10.9)	BSAD > PS***
Mixed affective episode	0	0	6 (2.7)	n.s.
Schizodepressive episode	6 (9.1)	0	39 (17.7)	ATPD > PS* BSAD > PS***
Schizomanic episode	2 (3.0)	0	32 (14.5)	BSAD > ATPD* BSAD > PS**
Mixed schizoaffective episode	2 (3.0)	0	15 (6.8)	BSAD > PS*
Schizophrenic episode	1 (1.5)	70 (94.5)	45 (20.5)	PS > ATPDS*** ATPD < BSAD*** BSAD < PS***
Other/not classifiable	8 (12.1)	3 (4.1)	18 (8.2)	n.s.

[a] Percentages in this table refer to all episodes before the index episode.
[b] Only pairwise comparisons with significant differences (χ^2 test or Fisher's exact test, two-tailed) are shown. * $P < 0.05$, ** $P < 0.01$, *** $P < 0.001$, n.s. no significance.

episodes were depressive, 9.1% schizodepressive, and 3% each manic, schizomanic and mixed schizoaffective. One ATPD patient had been treated at a different hospital for a schizophrenic episode more than 10 years earlier. After many years of remission, she had an acute episode of ATPD (F23.2, Acute Schizophrenia-like Psychotic Disorder) and was included in the study.

Patients with BSAD had a remarkably polymorphic course, as Table 7.2 shows. In contrast, the course of the schizophrenic patients was quite monomorphic. These issues are discussed in more detail in the following paragraphs that describe *the prospectively studied course.*

In the relapse analysis, all patients who had taken part in at least one prospective follow-up examination were included (ATPD $n = 39$, PS $n = 38$, BSAD $n = 37$). For each patient, the last available follow-up was defined as the end of the prospective observation period. This resulted in mean total prospective observation times of 4.6 years, 4.7 and 5.0 years for ATPD, PS and BSAD. All episodes of non-organic psychotic or non-organic major affective disorders that occurred during this period of time were defined as 'relapses' (see p. 62). Until the end of the prospective

Table 7.3. Frequency of relapses up to the end of the prospective follow-up time

	ATPD $n = 39$	PS $n = 38$	BSAD $n = 37$	
	n (%)	n (%)	n (%)	Statistical analysis[a]
Relapse until first follow-up	29 (76.3)	24 (63.4)	24 (64.9)	n.s.
Relapse during entire follow-up	30 (76.9)	29 (76.3)	28 (75.7)	n.s.
Number of relapses up to the end of the prospective follow-up (Mean ± SD)	1.6 ± 1.4	1.7 ± 2.1	2.0 ± 2.2	n.s.
Number of relapses up to the end of the prospective follow-up (range)	0–5	0–11	0–8	
	Mean ± SD	Mean ± SD	Mean ± SD	
Total prospective observation time	4.58 ± 1.51	4.69 ± 1.24	4.96 ± 1.35	n.s.
Annual frequency of episodes	0.37 ± 0.32	0.39 ± 0.48	0.38 ± 0.40	n.s.

[a] No significant differences in ANOVA or χ^2 test.

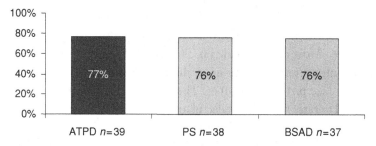

Fig. 7.1.   Proportion of patients with relapse up to the end of the prospective follow-up time.

follow-up, the majority of patients of all diagnostic groups had at least one relapse (up to 5 episodes for ATPD, up to 11 episodes for PS and up to 8 episodes for BSAD). As Fig. 7.1 shows, an almost equal number of patients in the three groups experienced relapses. Details on the number of relapses are given in Table 7.3. Although the maximum number of episodes was highest in the PS and BSAD groups, there was no significant difference between the three diagnostic groups regarding the total number of relapses up to the end of the prospective follow-up, or the number of relapses per year (annual frequency of episodes).

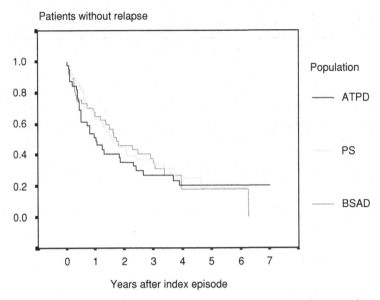

Fig. 7.2.   Kaplan–Meier analysis of the time to the first relapse after index episode.

Since the follow-up time varied between patients, a Kaplan–Meier survival analysis was calculated (Fig. 7.2). The mean time from index episode to relapse was 2.3 years for ATPD (95% confidence interval, 1.5–3.1 years), 2.5 years for PS (95% confidence interval, 1.8–3.2 years), and 2.5 years for BSAD (95% confidence interval, 1.7–3.2 years). There was no statistically significant difference in time from index episode to first relapse between the three groups (log rank test 0.58, d.f. = 2, $P = 0.749$). Most of the patients in the HASBAP were on continued medication (mostly antipsychotics), both upon discharge from the index admission, and at follow-up (see p. 164 and p. 166). The relapse rates found are rather high when compared to rates from controlled pharmacological trials (e.g. Gaebel *et al.*, 2002). The high relapse rate in the sample of the HASBAP, however, is consistent with a recent study by Robinson and co-workers (1999), who found a 5-year cumulative relapse rate of 81.9% in a sample of patients with first-episode schizophrenia or schizoaffective disorders who were carefully monitored by a dedicated research team and treated according to APA guidelines (Robinson *et al.*, 1999).

Conclusion: Relapse rates in Acute and Transient Psychotic Disorders are similar to those in controls with Positive Schizophrenia and Bipolar Schizoaffective Disorders. After 2.3 years, one-half of the Acute and Transient Psychotic Disorder patients will experience a relapse.

Table 7.4. Type of episode up to the end of the prospective follow-up time

ICD-10 episodes	ATPD $n = 63^a$ n (%)	PS $n = 65^a$ n (%)	BSAD $n = 75^a$ n (%)	Statistical analysis[b]
ATPD	35 (55.6)	4 (6.2)	4 (5.3)	ATPD > PS***
				ATPD > BSAD***
Depressive episode	16 (25.4)	3 (4.6)	23 (30.7)	ATPD > PS**
				BSAD > PS***
Manic episode	1 (1.6)	0	7 (9.3)	BSAD > PS*
Mixed affective episode	1 (1.6)	0	7 (9.3)	BSAD > PS*
All affective episodes	18 (28.6)	3 (4.6)	37 (49.3)	ATPD > PS***
				ATPD < BSAD*
				BSAD > PS***
Schizodepressive episode	4 (6.3)	1 (1.5)	14 (18.7)	ATPD < BSAD*
				PS < BSAD*
Schizomanic episode	0	0	8 (10.7)	ATPD < BSAD**
				PS < BSAD**
Mixed schizoaffective episode	2 (3.2)	0	5 (6.7)	n.s.
All schizoaffective episodes	6 (9.5)	1 (1.5)	27 (36.0)	BSAD > ATPD**
				BSAD > PS***
Schizophrenic episode	3 (4.8)	51 (78.5)	6 (8.0)	ATPD < PS***
				BSAD < PS***
Other/not classifiable	1 (1.6)	6 (9.2)	1 (1.3)	PS > BSAD*

[a] Numbers in this table refer to all episodes occurring between the index episode and the end of the prospective follow-up.
[b] Only pairwise comparisons with significant differences (χ^2 test or Fisher's exact test, two-tailed) are shown. $^*P < 0.05$, $^{**}P < 0.01$, $^{***}P < 0.001$, n.s. no significance.

Types of episode

Considerable interest concerns the question of what types of episode occur during the follow-up time. The answer to this question provides the basis for the discussion of diagnostic stability in ATPD and the control groups. In the HASBAP, ICD-10 diagnoses were assigned to every episode that occurred during the time from the index episode up to the end of the follow-up period. The procedure is analogous to the analysis of previous episodes (see also p. 63). Table 7.4. gives the results of this analysis. In the group of ATPD, the majority (55.6%) of the episodes occurring between the index episode and the end of the prospective follow-up also fulfilled the ICD-10 criteria of ATPD. Nevertheless, the remaining 44.4% of episodes were not ATPD episodes. Approximately 30% of them were affective episodes, especially depressive ones (25.4%), but schizoaffective and schizophrenic episodes occurred as well. Below, a distinction is introduced that is relevant to this topic.

The group of PS patients showed the greatest stability, with 78.5% of the episodes fulfilling the ICD-10 criteria of schizophrenia. Only 6% of the episodes during follow-up in the schizophrenic group fulfilled the criteria for a depressive episode, and only 1% of the episodes fulfilled the criteria for a schizodepressive one. Four episodes (6.2%) fulfilled the criteria for ATPD (three of these were episodes of Acute Schizophrenia-like Psychotic Disorder and one was ATPD, predominantly delusional).

The most frequent type of episode in the group of Bipolar Schizoaffective Disorders was affective episodes (49.5%), especially depressive episodes (30.7%), but also manic and mixed episodes (equally represented with 9.3%). Schizoaffective episodes were, with 36%, the second most frequent group of episodes. But also schizophrenic (8%) and ATPD (5.3%) occurred during the course of Bipolar Schizoaffective Disorders.

At this point, an important distinction has to be made. As is shown in more detail in Chapter 11, the subgroup of ATPD 'Schizophrenia-like Psychotic Disorders' (ICD-10 F23.2) seems to be distinct from the remaining ATPD and shows more similarities with typical schizophrenia. Therefore, it might be conceptually and methodologically more correct – in particular with regard to the stability of syndromes – to exclude this subcategory from the general category of ATPD. For this reason, the subgroup 'ATPD with Acute Schizophrenia-like Psychotic Disorder Excluded' was formed. The types of episodes during follow-up for this subgroup are given in Table 7.5. and contrasted with the results of the subgroup 'Acute Schizophrenia-like Psychotic Disorder'. There are now no schizophrenic episodes during the prospective follow-up time of 'ATPD-Acute Schizophrenia-like Psychotic Disorders Excluded'. When the new group of 'ATPD-Acute Schizophrenia-like Psychotic Disorders Excluded' is compared to the 'Acute Schizophrenia-like Psychotic Disorder', the subgroups differ from each other significantly, not only with regard to the occurrence of schizophrenic episodes, but also with regard to ATPD episodes which are more frequent in 'ATPD-Acute Schizophrenia-like Psychotic Disorders Excluded'.

Conclusion: Patients with Acute and Transient Psychotic Disorders who experience a relapse, usually have Acute and Transient Psychotic Disorder episodes again. Affective and schizoaffective episodes during follow-up, however, are also common.

Table 7.5. Type of episode up to the end of the prospective follow-up time in Acute Polymorphic Psychotic Disorder and Schizophrenia-like Psychotic Disorder[a]

ICD-10 episodes	ATPD (Acute Schizophrenia-like Psychosis excluded) $n = 43^a$	Acute Schizophrenia-like Psychosis $n = 20^a$	Statistical analysis[b]
	n (%)	n (%)	P
ATPD	29 (67.4)	6 (30.0)	0.005
Depressive episode	9 (20.9)	7 (35.0)	n.s.
Manic episode	1 (2.3)	0	n.s.
Mixed affective episode	1 (2.3)	0	n.s.
All affective episodes	11 (25.6)	7 (35.0)	n.s.
Schizodepressive episode	1 (2.3)	3 (15.0)	n.s.
Mixed schizoaffective episode	2 (4.7)	0	n.s.
Schizomanic episode	0	0	–
All schizoaffective episodes	3 (7.0)	3 (15.0)	n.s.
Schizophrenic episode	0	3 (15.0)	0.029[c]
Other/not classifiable	0	1 (5.0)	n.s.

[a] Numbers in this table refer to all episodes occurring between index episode and last point follow-up.

[b] χ^2 test, n.s. no significance.

[c] Fisher's exact test, two-tailed.

Diagnostic stability

From a theoretical point of view, one of the most important conditions for accepting separate entities in psychiatry is a strictly monomorphous course – or, in other words, a monosyndromal course, i.e. the occurrence of only one type of episode throughout the longitudinal course of the disorder. However, both clinical reality and longitudinal research demonstrate that the monosyndromal course is not the rule.

In the classical works of Karl Kahlbaum (1863, 1884), Emil Kraepelin (1896, 1920) and Eugen Bleuler (1911), the change of psychopathological syndromes during the course of psychotic disorders (syndrome shift) was described. The longitudinal studies conducted in Europe, and later also those conducted in America, confirmed these observations (Ciompi and Müller, 1976; Huber et al., 1979; Janzarik, 1968; Marneros et al., 1991b; Amin et al., 1999). Some authors reported a syndrome shift in more than 50% of the patients (Lewis and Pietrowski, 1954; Cutting et al., 1978; Horgan, 1981), but others found rates around 10% or even less (Clark and

Mallett, 1963; Angst *et al.*, 1978; Coryell and Winokur, 1980; Lee and Murray, 1988). But syndrome shift is dependent on the duration of observation time (Winokur *et al.*, 1985; Angst, 1986; Marneros *et al.*, 1988a, 1991b).

It seems that the group of schizophrenic patients has the highest stability of syndromes in the long term (Huber *et al.*, 1979; Janzarik 1968; Marneros *et al.*, 1991b,c). In a long-term investigation, the first author and his co-workers (the Cologne Study, Marneros *et al.*, 1991b), found that 90% of patients with an initial diagnosis of schizophrenia remained monomorphous (or monosyndromal) during a period of time of more than 25 years (i.e. they had only schizophrenic episodes). In contrast, schizoaffective disorders are longitudinally quite unstable (Marneros *et al.*, 1988a, 1991c). The stability of schizoaffective disorders in the long term seems to depend on the type of initial episode. Depressive and schizodepressive episodes show a remarkable stability of approximately 80%, while manic, schizomanic and mixed episodes only have a very weak syndrome stability (Marneros *et al.*, 1991c, 1995b). The low syndrome stability of Bipolar Schizoaffective Disorders found in our former studies (Marneros *et al.*, 1988c, 1991b,c, 1995b) was reconfirmed by the HASBAP.

Syndrome stability in ATPD, as defined by the WHO, has only rarely been studied. The cohort study of Amin and co-workers (1999) on diagnostic stability in first-episode psychosis included 30 patients with ICD-10 ATPD. After 3 years, 11 of these patients were still assigned a diagnosis of ATPD. Since in the study of Amin and co-workers (1999), apparently all who subsequently developed non-ATPD (e.g. affective) episodes were re-diagnosed at follow-up, the number of 11 patients would correspond to the ATPD with monosyndromal course in the HASBAP. Jørgensen and co-workers (1997) performed a 1-year follow-up on 51 patients with ICD-10 ATPD. They found a diagnostic shift in almost half of the patients (48%) – most often to affective disorder (28%) and schizophrenia (15%). However, only 33% of the patients had a relapse during the follow-up period. Hence, some of the diagnostic changes may have been the consequence of a different retrospective evaluation of the original episode at follow-up, rather than a result of the evolution of illness. It has been emphasised that diagnostic change due to 'measurement error' has to be differentiated from diagnostic change resulting from the evolution of the disorder ('real' syndrome shift) (Amin *et al.*, 1999).

In the following, the HASBAP findings are described in more detail. It has already been noted that 76.3% of all patients in the general group of ATPD had a relapse up to the end of the prospective follow-up time. After excluding Schizophrenia-like Psychoses, 78.6% of all patients with ATPD still had a relapse by the end of the prospective follow-up time – a virtually identical proportion (Fig. 7.3). Figure 7.4 shows how many of the patients who experienced a relapse had a monosyndromal or a polysyndromal course. A monosyndromal course is defined as a course during

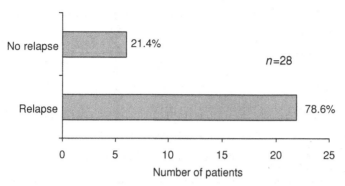

Fig. 7.3.   Number of subjects with relapse among ATPD (Acute Schizophrenia-like Psychoses excluded).

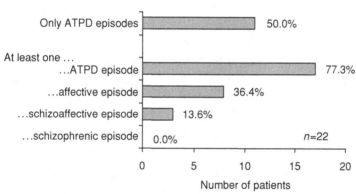

Fig. 7.4.   Monosyndromal versus polysyndromal course in ATPD (Acute Schizophrenia-like Psychoses excluded).

which only episodes of the same type as the index episode recur. A polysyndromal course must contain at least one other type of episode. As Fig. 7.4 shows, exactly one-half of patients with ATPD had only ATPD episodes (monosyndromal course). None of the patients had schizophrenic episodes, although a large majority of the patients had at least one ATPD episode (70%).

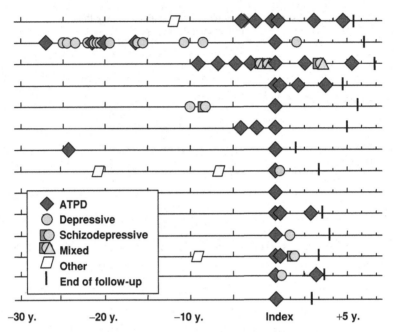

Fig. 7.5.   Syndrome shift in Acute Polymorphic Psychoses *Without* Symptoms of Schizophrenia (F23.0).

Following the ICD-10 subtyping of ATPD, the individual course of every patient was constructed according to the following subgroups:

1. 'Acute Polymorphic Psychoses Without Symptoms of Schizophrenia' (F23.0)
2. 'Acute Polymorphic Psychoses With Symptoms of Schizophrenia' (F23.1)
3. 'Acute Schizophrenia-like Psychoses' (F23.2)
4. 'ATPD, Predominantly Delusional, and Other' (F23.3/8).

Figures 7.5 to 7.8 show the detailed course for the individual patients of each subcategory. As is shown on the individual course diagram, none of the patients with 'Acute Polymorphic Psychoses *Without* Symptoms of Schizophrenia' developed a schizophrenic episode, but four of them experienced a depressive episode, one patient a schizodepressive episode and one a mixed schizoaffective episode (Fig. 7.5).

Patients with 'Acute Polymorphic Psychoses *With* Symptoms of Schizophrenia' did not develop schizophrenic episodes either (Fig. 7.6) until the end of the prospective follow-up period.

Four patients developed depressive episodes, while one developed a manic episode and two patients had schizoaffective episodes. *When the polymorphic groups were considered together, 60% of the patients with more than one episode had other kinds of episodes (especially affective and schizoaffective) than ATPD episodes during*

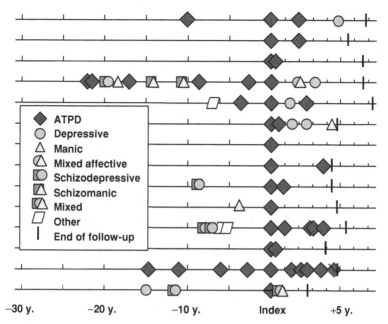

Fig. 7.6.   Syndrome shift in Acute Polymorphic Psychoses *With* Symptoms of Schizophrenia (F23.1).

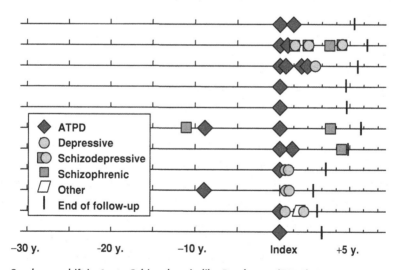

Fig. 7.7.   Syndrome shift in Acute Schizophrenia-like Psychoses (F23.2).

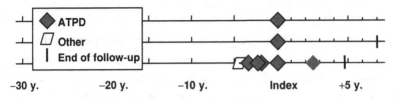

Fig. 7.8.   Syndrome shift in ATPD, Predominantly Delusional (F23.3) and Other ATPD (F23.8).

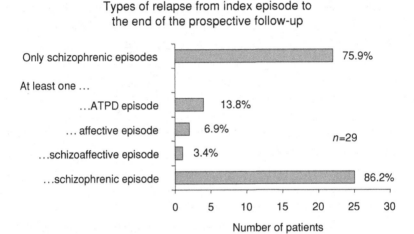

Fig. 7.9.   Monosyndromal vs. polysyndromal course in Positive Schizophrenia.

the entire course of the disorder (before and after the index episode) (see Tables 7.2 and 7.5.). The finding there were no schizophrenic episodes during the follow-up period in the two polymorphic groups is an additional argument that it might not be justified to separate the two groups (see p. 179ff).

In contrast, three of the eleven patients with an index diagnosis of 'Acute Schizophrenia-like Psychotic Disorder' developed episodes that fulfilled the ICD-10 criteria for schizophrenia. One patient with a schizophrenic episode also developed schizodepressive episodes. Only one patient with a relapse after the index episode showed exclusively ATPD episodes. Another four showed ATPD and depressive episodes. It seems that the group of Acute Schizophrenia-like Psychoses (F23.2) is the most problematic of the ATPD groups. The Schizophrenia-like Psychoses

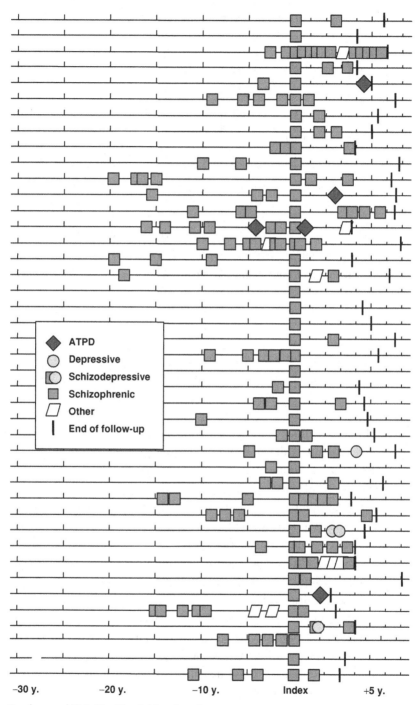

Fig. 7.10.   Syndrome shift in Positive Schizophrenia.

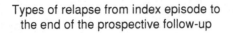

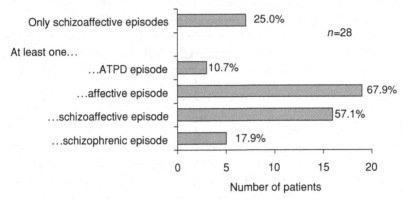

Percentages refer to all BSAD patients with a relapse.

Fig. 7.11.   Monosyndromal vs. polysyndromal course in Bipolar Schizoaffective Disorders.

subgroup does not belong to the ATPD group, but, rather a part of this group belongs to typical schizophrenia and another part belongs to the sequential form of schizoaffective disorder (Fig. 7.7).

Figure 7.8 shows the course diagrams of the subgroups ATPD F23.3 and F23.8 'ATPD, predominantly delusional' and 'other ATPD'. Two of the three patients could be followed-up, both had a monomorphous course.

Regarding *Schizophrenia*, the findings of the HASBAP are different from those regarding ATPD. As Fig. 7.9 shows, a large majority of schizophrenic patients (75.9%) had a monomorphous (monosyndromal) schizophrenic course. But nevertheless, 24.1% of the patients also experienced ATPD, affective or schizoaffective episodes. The following diagrams show the course of illness in individual patients with PS (Fig. 7.10). The Figures illustrate the predominance of schizophrenic episodes during the course of the group with PS and, therefore, the stability of schizophrenic disorders.

The *Bipolar Schizoaffective Disorders* are the most unstable of the three diagnostic groups. Only 25% of the patients had only schizoaffective episodes up to the end of the prospective follow-up period (Fig. 7.11). A large majority of them also had affective episodes, and some patients with schizophrenic episodes and ATPD episodes were also found.

The Proteus-like polysyndromal course of Bipolar Schizoaffective Disorders is also illustrated in Fig. 7.12.

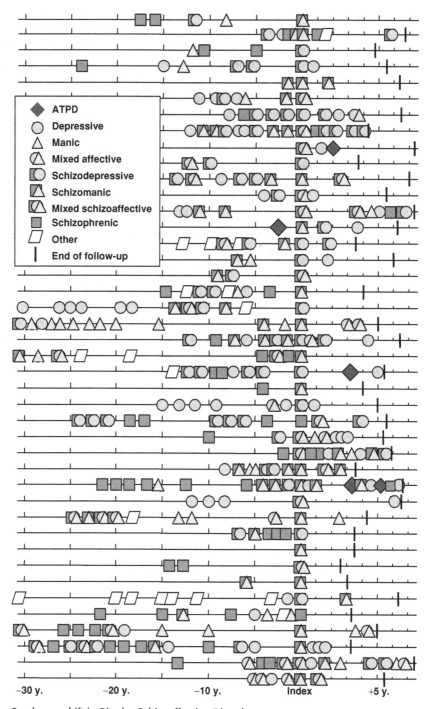

Fig. 7.12.　Syndrome shift in Bipolar Schizoaffective Disorders.

Conclusion: In the Halle Study on Brief and Acute Psychoses, instead of comparing 'overall' diagnoses at two different points in time, the sequence of syndromes in each individual patient is traced on the basis of all episodes that occurred up to the end of the prospective follow-up. Through this method, the syndrome stability of Acute and Transient Psychotic Disorders is found to be located in the middle between the high stability of schizophrenia and the low stability of schizoaffective disorder. In particular, after exclusion of the Acute Schizophrenia-like Psychotic Disorders from the group of Acute and Transient Psychotic Disorders, 50% of the Acute and Transient Psychotic Disorder patients have a 'monosyndromal' course during the prospective follow-up of five years (i.e. they are also diagnostically stable). This is compatible with the findings of the studies discussed above (Jørgensen et al., 1997; Amin et al., 1999). Yet, in the Halle Study on Brief and Acute Psychoses, one-half of the patients subsequently have, either additionally to Acute and Transient Psychotic Disorders or singularly, affective and schizoaffective episodes.

The high frequency of affective syndromes in the course of Acute and Transient Psychotic Disorders, fulfilling the criteria of depression, mania, or schizoaffective disorders, may indicate two, not mutually exclusive, possibilities: Firstly, a biological, especially genetic relationship between Acute and Transient Psychotic Disorders and affective disorders might exist – in a similar way as between schizoaffective and affective disorder (see overviews in Marneros and Tsuang, 1990). The second possible explanation is that Acute and Transient Psychotic Disorders constitute a 'bridge' between schizophrenia and depression. In other words, they have to be located on a continuum of affective and psychotic disorders (Marneros et al., 1995b; Crow, 1995, 2000; Angst and Marneros, 2001).

8

The long-term outcome

When, in this chapter, the 'outcome' of the disorders investigated is described, it has to be borne in mind that the term 'outcome' is a difficult and problematic term (Strauss and Carpenter, 1972; Marneros *et al.*, 1991b; Davidson and McGlashan, 1997; Riecher-Rössler and Rössler, 1998). Any single definition of 'outcome' must be arbitrary for two reasons. Firstly, the outcome of a mental disorder as something unchangeable and definitive only rarely exists. It would be incorrect to connect the notion of outcome with something 'final' and 'unchangeable' since alterations in psychopathological and social status, changes in psychological and social functioning, remission or deterioration are always possible during life. The term outcome is therefore only a compromise describing the status of the patient at a point following a period of time after the onset of illness (Marneros *et al.*, 1990c). Secondly, the term outcome has various meanings (e.g. it may refer to persisting psychopathological symptoms or symptom-free periods, to the presence or absence of disability, to persisting alterations of personality, or to restrictions of the patient's social status or functioning). There is no favourable or unfavourable outcome, but there is a continuum between 'full health' and 'full disability'. In psychiatric populations, both ends of the continuum are the exception rather than the rule. In this sense, in the following chapters, various aspects of 'outcome' are described, including global functioning, disability, psychological impairment, autarky, persisting symptomatology, interpersonal relations, etc.

A favourable long-term outcome as the rule is an important feature of all the predecessors of ATPD, although some modifications apply. Perris (1974), in his landmark study on cycloid psychoses, found that some of these patients received invalidity pensions because frequent relapses made paid work impossible, and in a few patients, the intervals became so short that these patients had to be considered as chronically ill. In most patients, however, no psychopathology was noticed at follow-up. Brockington and co-workers (1982a), in their retrospective study of 30 patients with cycloid psychoses, found complete recovery in 92% (compared to 59% in the general group of patients with endogenous psychoses). Kimura and co-workers (1980) investigated patients with atypical psychoses and found light or medium residual syndromes in 19 of 58 patients, but even in the 19 patients with residual symptoms, they were qualitatively different from the typical schizophrenic residuum. In 1986 Singer and co-workers (Singer *et al.*, 1986) conducted a follow-up study on 43 patients who had been treated in 1972 for bouffée délirante, and on a comparison group of 72 patients with schizophrenia. At follow-up, significantly more patients with schizophrenia than with bouffée délirante were unable to work. Social recovery was found in 10 of 44 patients with schizophrenia, but in 11 of 26 patients with bouffée délirante. An unfavourable course was present in 18 of 44 patients with schizophrenia and 5 of 26 patients with bouffée délirante. Follow-up investigations with internationally recognised scales of patients with cycloid psychoses were reported by Maj (1988, 1990a) and Beckmann and co-workers (1990). These studies confirmed a relatively favourable course of cycloid psychoses.

Apart from the HASBAP, the only prospective studies giving differentiated follow-up data on a cohort of patients with ATPD are the investigation by Jørgensen (1997), and, to a limited degree, by Sajith and co-workers (2002). These data are mentioned below.

The HASBAP investigated the outcome of ATPD in terms of functional, psychopathological and social status. The basis of this data is the second follow-up interview conducted at the end of the prospective follow-up period. For assessment of the above-mentioned aspects, the instruments mentioned in Table 3.1 and described in detail on page 56ff were applied. The mean duration of illness at the end of the prospective follow-up was 10.2 years for ATPD, 10.8 years for PS and 17.8 years for BSAD. The mean time that had elapsed since the index episode was 4.8 years for ATPD, 5.0 years for PS and 5.2 years for BSAD (see Table 3.2).

Global functioning at the end of the prospective follow-up period

In his follow-up study on retrospectively diagnosed patients with ATPD, Jørgensen (1995) reported a mean GAS score of 70 at the 8-year follow-up. Jørgensen and co-workers (1997) reported an identical mean value of 70 for 24 ATPD patients at the 1-year follow-up. It should be noted that this value refers to the 24 of initially 51 patients who at follow-up were still believed to belong to the diagnostic category of ATPD.

Sajith and co-workers (2002), in their study of 45 patients with Acute Polymorphic Psychotic Disorder in Pondicherry, India, reported a mean GAS score of 68.8 after 3 years and a standard deviation of 8.7. The GAS score of those patients retaining a diagnosis of Acute Polymorphic Psychotic Disorder after 3 years was

Table 8.1. Global Assessment Scale scores at the end of the prospective follow-up period

	ATPD	PS	BSAD	
	$n = 38$	$n = 34$	$n = 34$	Statistical analysis
GAS score[b]				
Mean ± SD	81.7 ± 15.3	61.8 ± 21.7	78.3 ± 11.2	$P < 0.001$[a]
				ATPD > PS***
				BSAD > PS***
Range	30–98	25–95	42–97	
Level of functioning	n (%)	n (%)	n (%)	
Good (71–100)	31 (81.6)	12 (35.3)	25 (73.5)	ATPD > PS*** [c]
				BSAD > PS**
Medium (51–70)	5 (13.2)	11 (32.4)	8 (23.5)	n.s.
Severely impaired (31–50)	1 (2.6)	8 (23.5)	1 (2.9)	ATPD > PS*
				BSAD < PS*
Most severely impaired (<30)	1 (2.6)	3 (8.8)	0	n.s.

[a] ANOVA: pairwise comparisons with significant differences (Scheffé procedure) are indicated.
[b] Possible scores range from 0 to 100, higher score indicating better functioning.
[c] Only pairwise comparisons with significant differences (χ^2 test or Fisher's exact test, two-tailed) are shown.
*$P < 0.05$, **$P < 0.01$, ***$P < 0.001$, n.s. no significance.

significantly higher (71.5 ± 4.8) than that of those patients with a diagnostic change (61.1 ± 12.3).

The findings of the HASBAP are shown in Table 8.1. Although a wide range of GAS scores can be found in all three groups, the mean scores clearly show that the overall functioning of the ATPD patients was significantly better than that of patients with PS. ATPD patients, however, did not differ significantly from the BSAD group in terms of mean scores. Comparing the rate of patients with a GAS score greater than 70 ('good functioning'), it was found that almost 82% of patients with ATPD showed good functioning, which is significantly more frequent than in the group of schizophrenia (35%). Again, there was no difference between ATPD patients and patients with BSAD (74%) regarding 'good functioning'.

Conclusion: Patients with Acute and Transient Psychotic Disorders have the most favourable outcome in comparison to the other psychotic patients. Additionally, in contrast to schizophrenic patients, patients with Acute and Transient Psychotic Disorders or Bipolar Schizoaffective Disorders only rarely show severe (scores lower than 51) or very severe (scores lower than 31) levels of impairment.

Table 8.2. WHO/DAS scores at the end of the prospective follow-up period

	ATPD $n = 38$	PS $n = 34$	BSAD $n = 34$	
	Mean ± SD	Mean ± SD	Mean ± SD	Statistical analysis
DAS Global score[c]	0.58 ± 1.00	1.97 ± 1.42	0.85 ± 0.82	$P < 0.001^a$ ATPD < PS*** BSAD < PS***
DAS General behaviour subscore[c]	0.55 ± .92	1.55 ± 1.22	0.66 ± 0.63	$P < 0.001^a$ ATPD < PS*** BSAD < PS***
DAS Special roles subscore[c]	0.89 ± 1.09	2.18 ± 1.52	1.45 ± 0.89	$P < 0.001^a$ ATPD < PS*** BSAD < PS*
	n (%)	n (%)	n (%)	
Good social functioning (Score 0)	25 (65.8)	6 (17.6)	12 (35.3)	ATPD > PS*** [b] ATPD > BSAD**
Sufficient social functioning (Score 1)	8 (21.1)	9 (26.5)	17 (50.0)	ATPD < BSAD* PS < BSAD*
Moderate social functioning (Score 2)	2 (5.3)	6 (17.6)	3 (8.8)	n.s.
Low social functioning (Score 3)	2 (5.3)	6 (17.6)	2 (5.9)	n.s.
Bad social functioning (Score 4)	1 (2.6)	7 (20.6)	0	PS > BSAD*
Absent social functioning (Score 5)	0	0	0	–

[a] ANOVA: pairwise comparisons with significant differences (Scheffé procedure) are indicated.
[b] Only pairwise comparisons with significant differences (χ^2 test or Fisher's exact test, two-tailed) are shown.
* $P < 0.05$, ** $P < 0.01$, *** $P < 0.001$, n.s. no significance.
[c] Possible scores range from 0 to 5, higher score indicating greater deficit.

Social disability according to WHO criteria

The instrument used to assess disability was the WHO Disability Assessment Schedule (WHO/DAS). Table 8.2 reports WHO/DAS scores at the end of the prospective follow-up period as a measure of disability. The lowest WHO/DAS scores (indicating least disability) were found in patients with ATPD who differed significantly from PS patients who showed the highest scores. Although differences also emerged between ATPD and BSAD, they did not reach a significant level. However, when looking at patients scoring 0 (i.e. good social functioning), it could be found that significantly more patients with ATPD (66%) than schizophrenic (18%) and schizoaffective (35%) patients, had good social functioning.

Table 8.3. WHO/DAS at the end of the prospective follow-up period: patients with disability in particular domains

	ATPD $n = 38$	PS $n = 34$	BSAD $n = 34$	Statistical analysis[a]
	n (%)	n (%)	n (%)	P
Partner relationship	17 (44.7)	26 (76.5)	21 (61.8)	ATPD < PS**
Work role[b]	16 (48.5)	24 (82.8)	30 (90.9)	ATPD < PS**
				ATPD < BSAD**
Social withdrawal	13 (34.2)	23 (67.6)	11 (32.4)	ATPD < PS**
				BSAD < PS**
Household participation	6 (15.8)	17 (50.0)	11 (32.4)	ATPD < PS**
General interests	8 (21.1)	16 (47.1)	9 (26.5)	ATPD < PS**
Self-care	4 (10.5)	18 (52.9)	4 (11.8)	ATPD < PS***
				PS > BSAD***
Social friction	3 (7.9)	8 (23.5)	6 (17.6)	n.s.

[a] Only pairwise comparisons with significant differences (χ^2 test or Fisher's exact test, two-tailed) are shown. ** $P < 0.01$, *** $P < 0.001$, n.s. no significance.
[b] All patients aged 60 or older excluded (different n: ATPD 33, PS 29, BSAD 33).

The WHO/DAS global score as well as the subscores 'general behaviour' and 'special roles' are highly aggregated measures that cannot easily be related to concrete domains of social functioning. To better understand which particular domains of social functioning were disturbed, a method suggested by Wiersma and co-workers (2000) was employed to break down the WHO/DAS items into seven categories. Each of these categories refers to a particular domain of social functioning (partner relationship, work role, social withdrawal, household participation, general interests, self-care, social friction). Table 8.3 gives the numbers and proportions of patients in each group who have disabilities in the respective domains. It becomes clear from Table 8.3 that different domains are not affected equally. Group differences are greatest in self-care where a high proportion of PS is impaired, but very few patients with ATPD or BSAD. A similar pattern exists with regard to social withdrawal and general interests. With regard to partner relationship, household participation and social friction, the number of impaired patients in BSAD appears to be higher than in ATPD, but lower than in PS, although for some comparisons, the numbers are too small for statistical significance. This is especially true for social friction, which was rare in all samples. The work role was exceptionally frequently disturbed in PS and BSAD patients. The reasons for this are discussed below.

Table 8.4. PANSS scores at the end of the prospective follow-up period

	ATPD $n = 38$	PS $n = 33$	BSAD $n = 34$	
	Mean ± SD	Mean ± SD	Mean ± SD	Statistical analysis[a]
PANSS Positive Subscale[b]	8.1 ± 3.2	10.4 ± 5.7	7.8 ± 1.5	$P = 0.012$ ATPD < PS* BSAD < PS*
PANSS Negative Subscale[b]	10.5 ± 6.2	17.1 ± 9.1	10.2 ± 5.3	$P < 0.001$ ATPD < PS** BSAD < PS**
PANSS General Subscale[b]	19.5 ± 6.3	24.3 ± 7.4	19.5 ± 3.6	$P = 0.001$ ATPD < PS* BSAD < PS*
PANSS Total Scale[b]	38.1 ± 14.0	51.8 ± 19.7	37.5 ± 8.3	$P < 0.001$ ATPD < PS** BSAD < PS**

[a] ANOVA, only significant differences in *post-hoc* Scheffé tests given, $*P < 0.05$, $**P < 0.01$.
[b] Possible scores range from 7–49 for positive and negative subscale, from 16 to 112 on the general subscale and from 30 to 210 on the total scale, higher score indicating more symptoms.

> Conclusion: Two-thirds of patients with Acute and Transient Psychotic Disorders had, at the end of the prospective follow-up period, a good social functioning according to WHO/DAS and therefore a more favourable outcome than patients with schizophrenia and schizoaffective disorders.

Psychopathological outcome

The psychopathological outcome was estimated by:
(a) *assessment of symptoms using the PANSS* and
(b) estimating *persisting alterations*.

Assessment of symptoms using the PANSS

With the Positive and Negative Syndrome Scale (PANSS, Kay *et al.*, 1989), present state psychopathological symptoms in psychotic disorders can be reliably assessed (see p. 66). The PANSS is used widely in psychiatric research and allows for the differentiation of a positive and a negative syndrome. Additionally, there is a score for general symptomatology and a total score. PANSS scores in the samples of the HASBAP, referring to the end of the prospective follow-up, are given in Table 8.4.

Table 8.5. Persisting alterations at the end of the prospective follow-up period

	ATPD $n = 38$	PS $n = 33$	BSAD $n = 34$	
	n (%)	n (%)	n (%)	Statistical analysis[a]
No persisting alterations	27 (71.1)	7 (21.2)	19 (55.9)	APTD > PS*** BSAD > PS**
Slight asthenic-insufficiency syndrome	5 (13.2)	6 (18.2)	11 (32.4)	n.s.
Adynamic-deficient syndrome	4 (10.5)	10 (30.3)	4 (11.8)	APTD < PS*
Depletion syndrome	0	2 (6.1)	0	n.s.
Apathetic paranoid syndrome (or apathetic-hallucinatory syndrome)	2 (5.3)	1 (3.0)	0	n.s.
Chronic psychosis	0	6 (18.2)	0	APTD > PS** BSAD > PS*
Structural deformation of personality	0	1 (3.0)	0	n.s.

[a] Only pairwise comparisons with significant differences (χ^2 test or Fisher's exact test, two-tailed) are shown. *$P < 0.05$, **$P < 0.01$, ***$P < 0.001$, n.s. no significance.

There were essentially no differences in PANSS scores between BSAD and ATPD patients at the end of the prospective follow-up. As can be seen in Table 8.4, mean symptom scores for both groups were very near the baseline of the scale. In contrast, patients with PS showed significantly higher (more pathological) scores than both ATPD and BSAD. The higher symptom scores of the PS patients were seen on all scales, but they were particularly prominent on the negative syndrome scale.

> Conclusion: Patients with Acute and Transient Psychotic Disorder, as well as Bipolar Schizoaffective Disorder, show very little present state symptomatology at the end of the prospective follow-up, both in terms of positive and negative symptoms. They differ significantly from the patients with Positive Schizophrenia, in whom negative symptoms in particular are much more frequent.

Persisting alterations (residual syndrome)

Presence and type of persisting alterations were assessed by definitions and criteria described on page 67. Table 8.5 gives the number of patients with persisting alterations at the end of the prospective follow-up. The majority of ATPD patients were free from persisting alterations (71.1%). Five patients (13.2%) showed a slight asthenic-insufficiency syndrome (see Marneros and Rohde, 1997; Marneros *et al.*, 1998). Alterations of these kind are unspecific (e.g. in the Cologne study, a slight asthenic-insufficiency syndrome was found in 20.8% of 106 patients with affective disorders after long-term course) (Marneros *et al.*, 1991b). The adynamic-deficient syndrome (found in 10.5% of the ATPD patients) still represents a less severe phenomenology of persisting alterations. Only two patients from the ATPD group (5.3%) showed a severe phenomenological type of persisting alteration, namely an apathetic paranoid syndrome involving persisting delusions and hallucinations and severe disturbance of drive and affect.

In contrast, persisting alterations in PS at the end of the prospective follow-up were both significantly more frequent than in ATPD and, in many patients, took a more severe form, in particular that of chronic psychosis. Persisting alterations in BSAD, although significantly more frequent than in ATPD, did not differ in the phenomenological types.

Conclusion: Although 28.9% of the patients with Acute and Transient Psychotic Disorders develop persisting alterations during the course of illness, the persisting alterations usually are of less severe form. In this regard, patients with Acute and Transient Psychotic Disorder, as well as patients with Bipolar Schizoaffective Disorder, differ significantly from the group with Positive Schizophrenia, in whom severe persisting alterations are more frequent.

Social consequences

Employment status

Employment status is a very sensitive parameter of long-term outcome. When Jørgensen and co-workers (1997) reported clinical and social functioning at the 1-year follow-up in their cohort of 51 patients with ATPD, the subscale 'employment' showed the lowest value of the four subscales of the McGlashan outcome scale (the others being hospitalisation, social contacts and psychopathology). Similar findings emerged in the HASBAP regarding disability payments due to the psychotic disorder, as Table 8.6 shows. At the end of the prospective follow-up period, the ATPD patients showed the highest rate of employment of all clinical groups. However, the most impressive finding in this analysis is the high proportion of patients with disability pension especially in the group of PS and BSAD. Less than 15% of patients with BSAD and less than 30% of the patients with PS were

Table 8.6. Employment status at the end of the prospective follow-up period

	ATPD $n = 38$	PS $n = 34$	BSAD $n = 34$	
	n (%)	n (%)	n (%)	Statistical analysis[a]
Disability pension[b]	14 (36.8)	24 (70.6)	29 (85.3)	ATPD < PS**
				ATPD < BSAD***
Unemployed	8 (21.1)	2 (5.9)	1 (2.9)	ATPD > BSAD*
Employed	11 (28.9)	5 (14.7)	3 (8.8)	ATPD > BSAD*
Old age pension	2 (5.3)	2 (5.9)	0	n.s.
Vocational training	3 (7.9)	1 (2.9)	1 (2.9)	n.s.

[a] Only pairwise comparisons with significant differences (χ^2 test or Fisher's exact test, two-tailed) are shown. *$P < 0.05$, **$P < 0.01$, ***$P < 0.001$, n.s. no significance.
[b] One ATPD patient received disability pension because of somatic disease, all others because of the psychiatric disorder.

without a disability pension. There was no statistical significant difference between PS and BSAD. Although significantly more patients with ATPD were without disability pensions, the proportion of patients receiving a disability pension (almost 40%) is very high when the relatively good functional level of the ATPD patients is considered. Most likely, these findings reflect a sociopolitical reality: due to the structural weakness of the former political system, unemployment in East Germany after reunification is very high (in the city of Halle it amounts to more than 20%). Hence, patients with mental illness, independent of their level of functioning, have many more difficulties getting a job than mentally healthy people. This could be an explanation for why the political authorities tend to relatively easily grant a disability pension to mentally ill people. Vice versa, people with mental problems and difficulties in occupational life, especially with regard to finding a job, tend to apply for a disability pension in order to avoid the negative consequences of unemployment.

> Conclusion: The employment status of patients with Acute and Transient Psychotic Disorders at the end of the prospective follow-up period is significantly better than that of schizophrenic and bipolar schizoaffective patients.

Stable heterosexual relationship

It is well established that patients with schizophrenia show reduced rates of marriage and long-term heterosexual relationships when compared to demographically

Table 8.7. Stable heterosexual relationship at the end of the prospective follow-up period

	ATPD $n = 38$	PS $n = 34$	BSAD $n = 34$	
	n (%)	n (%)	n (%)	Statistical analysis[a]
With partner	24 (63.2)	13 (38.2)	17 (50.0)	ATPD > PS*
Without partner	14 (36.8)	21 (61.8)	17 (50.0)	

[a] Only pairwise comparisons with significant differences (χ^2 test or Fisher's exact test, two-tailed) are shown. *$P < 0.05$.

similar controls (Eaton, 1975; Watt and Szulecka, 1979; Riecher-Rössler et al., 1992; Tsuang et al., 1995; Thara and Srinivasan, 1997). The difference occurs early in the course of illness (Riecher-Rössler et al., 1992), is more prominent in men than in women (Watt and Szulecka, 1979), and appears to be associated with an unfavourable course (Tien and Eaton, 1992). Although a protective influence of marriage and stable relationships has been discussed (Eaton, 1975), most evidence indicates that either interactional deficits or premorbid personality features associated with schizophrenia are responsible for the low rates of marriage and partnership in schizophrenia (Watt and Szulecka, 1979; Riecher-Rössler et al., 1992; Thara and Srinivasan, 1997).

Jönsson and co-workers (1991) found higher rates of marriage in a historical cohort of cycloid patients than in controls with schizophrenia, both pre- and postmorbidly. In the HASBAP, fewer patients from the ATPD group had a stable heterosexual relationship before onset than patients from the PS group, but ATPD patients did not differ from healthy controls in that respect (see p. 92). Table 8.7 shows the number of patients with a stable heterosexual relationship at the end of the prospective follow-up. At the end of the prospective follow-up period, the majority of patients with ATPD had a stable heterosexual relationship (63%). This is nearly the same number as was found at the first follow-up point approximately 3 years earlier. In contrast, significantly fewer patients with schizophrenia had a stable heterosexual relationship (35%) as was the case with the first point of follow-up. Although, with regard of to the group with Bipolar Schizoaffective Disorder, the proportion with a stable relationship at the end of the prospective follow-up period was somewhat reduced in comparison to the first follow-up, this difference was negligible, even when considering the three drop-outs at the end of the prospective follow-up period.

Table 8.8. Autarky at the end of the prospective follow-up period

	ATPD $n = 38$	PS $n = 34$	BSAD $n = 34$	
	n (%)	n (%)	n (%)	Statistical analysis[a]
Full autarky	34 (89.5)	20 (58.8)	30 (88.2)	ATPD > PS**
				BSAD > PS**
No autarky, not in institution	3 (7.9)	9 (26.5)	4 (11.8)	PS > ATPD*
No autarky, permanently in institution	1 (2.6)	5 (14.7)		n.s.

[a] Only pairwise comparisons with significant differences (χ^2 test or Fisher's exact test, two-tailed) are shown. *$P < 0.05$, **$P < 0.01$, n.s. no significance.

> Conclusion: Throughout the course of illness, patients with Acute and Transient Psychotic Disorders, but also Bipolar Schizoaffective patients, show rates of stable heterosexual relationship that are similar to those of healthy controls. In contrast, in schizophrenia the number of patients with stable relationships is reduced even before the onset of the disorder. The difference between Acute and Transient Psychotic Disorders and schizophrenia stays significant up to the end of the prospective follow-up.

Autarky

Autarky is defined as the capability of independent living with or without giving support to other family members (Marneros *et al.*, 1991a). Table 8.8 gives the numbers of patients with and without autarky at the end of the prospective follow-up period. Only four patients from the groups Acute and Transient Psychotic Disorders and Bipolar Schizoaffective Disorders had lost their autarky at the end of the prospective follow-up – this is significantly less than the number of patients with PS who had lost their autarky. The one ATPD patient who was institutionalised at the end of the prospective follow-up had developed a severe schizophrenic episode during this time after which he had to be referred to an institution.

> Conclusion: Loss of autarky is rare in both Acute and Transient Psychotic Disorders and Bipolar Schizoaffective Disorder compared to schizophrenia. These findings again support the better prognosis of Acute and Transient Psychotic Disorders and Bipolar Schizoaffective Disorder in comparison with schizophrenia.

Table 8.9. Highest socio-economic status (SES) achieved

	ATPD $n = 42$	PS $n = 42$	BSAD $n = 42$	CNTR $n = 42$	
	n (%)	n (%)	n (%)	n (%)	Statistical analysis[a]
Highest SES achieved					ATPD > PS**
					CNTR > PS*
Very high SES	2 (4.8)	1 (2.4)	1 (2.4)	1 (2.4)	
High SES	12 (28.6)	3 (7.1)	7 (16.7)	10 (23.8)	
Medium SES	8 (19.0)	6 (14.3)	7 (16.7)	9 (21.4)	
Low SES	15 (35.7)	21 (50.0)	23 (54.8)	17 (40.5)	
Very low SES	5 (11.9)	9 (21.4)	4 (9.5)	4 (9.5)	
Unclassifiable		2 (4.8)		1 (2.4)	

SES Socio-economic status.
[a] Only pairwise comparisons with significant differences (Mann-Whitney U-test) are shown.
*$P < 0.05$, **$P < 0.01$.

Socio-economic status

The theoretical background and rationale for the evaluation of socio-economic status (SES) were discussed above (p. 89). It was shown that patients of the PS group had a lower socio-economic status (SES) than ATPD patients at the onset of the disorder, although there was no difference in SES of the families of origin.

At both follow-up points, the occupational history during the period of follow-up was assessed. On the basis of the data from all time points, the highest SES achieved during the lifetime of all of the patients and mentally healthy controls was calculated according to the criteria detailed on page 90. Table 8.9 gives the results of this evaluation. It becomes clear from this table that patients with PS did not reach the same socio-economic level as patients with ATPD and mentally healthy controls. There were no significant differences between ATPD, BSAD and mentally healthy controls.

Social mobility with respect to the family of origin is reported Table 8.10. Patients or subjects with a higher SES than their families of origin can be said to have experienced upward social mobility, while patients or subjects with a lower SES than their families of origin have experienced downward social mobility, and patients or subjects with SES equal to that of their families of origin can be regarded as socially stable. Again, this analysis reveals an underachievement of patients with Positive Schizophrenia that becomes significant both in comparison to ATPD and to Bipolar Schizoaffective Disorder.

Table 8.10. Social mobility: subjects' highest SES achieved compared with SES of family of origin

	ATPD $n = 40$	PS $n = 37$	BSAD $n = 40$	CNTR $n = 40$	
	n (%)	n (%)	n (%)	n (%)	Statistical analysis[a]
Lower SES	10 (25.0)	17 (45.9)	12 (30.0)	8 (20.0)	CNTR > PS*
Equal SES	13 (32.5)	13 (35.1)	17 (42.5)	18 (45.0)	n.s.
Higher SES	17 (42.5)	7 (18.9)	11 (27.5)	14 (35.0)	ATPD > PS*

SES Socio-economic status.

[a] Only pairwise comparisons with significant differences (χ^2 test or Fisher's exact test, two-tailed) are shown. * $P < 0.05$, n.s. no significance.

Conclusion: The findings on socio-economic status confirm the numerous reports in the literature of increased downward social mobility in schizophrenia (Goldberg and Morrison, 1963; Wiersma et al., 1983; Eaton, 1985; Angermeyer and Klusmann, 1987; Jones et al., 1993). However, in Acute and Transient Psychotic Disorders and in Bipolar Schizoaffective Disorder, no significant difference in social mobility can be found to mentally healthy controls.

Summary and conclusion from findings on outcome

Conclusion: On a wide range of standardised rating scales and psychosocial indicators of outcome, significant differences between the investigated groups emerge. The clearest and most consistent differences exist between Acute and Transient Psychotic Disorders and the group with schizophrenia. After 10 years of illness, patients with Acute and Transient Psychotic Disorder show (in comparison to controls with schizophrenia) better global functioning, less social disability, fewer persisting alterations, fewer negative, as well as fewer positive, symptoms and higher rates of heterosexual relationships. In most aspects of outcome, patients with Acute and Transient Psychotic Disorder as a group do not differ from mentally healthy controls, although they are significantly impaired in their occupational status when compared to the mentally healthy subjects. Moreover, in a small minority of Acute and Transient Psychotic Disorder patients, unfavourable outcome states occur including severely impaired global functioning and loss of autarky. Patients with Bipolar Schizoaffective Disorder are very similar to patients with Acute and Transient Psychotic Disorders in many aspects of outcome, but do not reach the level of mentally healthy controls (e.g. in terms of global functioning, psychological impairment and autarky). Patients with Bipolar Schizoaffective Disorder also differ significantly from patients with Acute and Transient Psychotic Disorder in showing much higher rates of disability pension at follow-up. The Halle Study on Brief and Acute Psychoses data on the outcome of Acute and Transient Psychotic Disorders are in accordance with the findings on Acute and Transient Psychotic Disorders of Jørgensen and co-workers (1997) in Denmark and of Sajith and co-workers (2002) in their Indian study. These data are also consistent with earlier studies demonstrating a favourable outcome of cycloid psychoses in comparison to schizophrenia and schizoaffective psychoses (Maj, 1988, 1990a; Beckmann et al., 1990). While, again, outcome cannot be described as monolithic, the bulk of the data discussed here indicate that outcome in Acute and Transient Psychotic Disorders is clearly more favourable than in schizophrenia, but only slightly more favourable than in Bipolar Schizoaffective Disorder.

9

Suicidal behaviour

Suicidal behaviour is an important and frequent phenomenon not only in affective disorders, but also in schizophrenia and schizoaffective disorders (Angst and Clayton, 1986; Marneros *et al.*, 1991b; Gupta *et al.*, 1998; Tsuang *et al.*, 1999). Completed suicide is the most disastrous outcome of psychiatric disorders. While a good deal of research has been conducted on suicidal behaviour in affective disorders and schizophrenia (Tsuang *et al.*, 1999; Hawton and Van Heeringen, 2000), suicidality in ATPD has not yet been investigated. The HASBAP is the first study addressing the issue of suicidality in ATPD.

In this chapter, the findings of the HASBAP on suicidal behaviour in ATPD and the clinical control groups are reported. Data on suicidal behaviour were collected during the sociobiographical interview and supplemented by the analysis of hospital records. For every patient who died during the follow-up period, information was collected from sources to verify the cause and the circumstances of death.

In the acute episode, the frequency of suicidal symptoms (including suicidal ideation and suicide attempts) was highest in ATPD patients (26.2%), followed by BSAD (23.8%) and PS patients (11.9%). Frequency of suicidal ideation differed non-significantly between diagnostic groups. Suicide attempts during the acute episode were, in the sample of the HASBAP, only observed in ATPD and BSAD (Table 9.1). The difference between ATPD and PS was highly significant. Closer examination of the suicide attempts showed that in ATPD, all suicide attempts happened at a maximum of two days before admission, while in BSAD, suicide attempts happened between one day and eight weeks before the presence of full clinical symptomatology. It is likely that the close temporal connection of the suicide attempts to the psychotic symptoms in ATPD reflects the acuity and the turmoil of the clinical picture. Table 9.2 gives the frequency of suicide attempts *during the whole course of illness* and also the number of patients who committed suicide during the period of follow-up. The frequency of suicidal behaviour was high in all groups. In ATPD, suicidal behaviour during the *whole course* of the illness (mean duration 10.2 years) was found in 35.7% of the patients, but none of them

Table 9.1. Frequency of suicidal ideation and suicide attempts in the acute episode

	ATPD $n = 42$	PS $n = 42$	BSAD $n = 42$	
	n (%)	n (%)	n (%)	Statistical analysis[a]
Suicidal symptoms	11 (26.2)	5 (11.9)	10 (23.8)	n.s.
Suicidal ideation	3 (7.1)	5 (11.9)	5 (11.9)	n.s.
Suicide attempts	8 (19.0)	0	5 (11.9)	ATPD > PS**

[a] Only pairwise comparisons with significant differences (χ^2 test or Fisher's exact test, two-tailed) are shown. ** $P < 0.01$, n.s. no significance.

Table 9.2. Frequency of suicidal behaviour during the whole course of the illness

	ATPD $n = 42$	PS $n = 42$	BSAD $n = 42$	
	n (%)	n (%)	n (%)	Statistical analysis[a]
Suicidal behaviour in general	15 (35.7)	17 (40.5)	24 (57.1)	ATPD < BSAD*
Suicide attempts	15 (35.7)	15 (35.7)	21 (50.0)	n.s.
One	6 (14.3)	8 (19.0)	7 (16.7)	n.s.
More than one	9 (21.4)	7 (16.7)	14 (33.3)	n.s.
Committed suicide	0	2 (4.8)	3 (7.1)	n.s.

[a] Only pairwise comparisons with significant differences (χ^2 test or Fisher's exact test, two-tailed) are shown. * $P < 0.05$, n.s. no significance.

committed suicide (Table 9.2). In Positive Schizophrenia, the proportion of patients with suicidal behaviour during the whole course of the illness (mean duration 10.8 years) was found to be 40.5%. One female and one male schizophrenic patient committed suicide during the follow-up period. The highest rate of suicidal behaviour during the longitudinal course (mean duration 17.8 years) was observed in BSAD (57.1%). Three of the BSAD patients (two male, one female) committed suicide during follow-up. Among those patients who attempted suicide, the number of suicide attempts varied between one and eight. In BSAD, the overall frequency of suicidal behaviour was highest and the difference to ATPD reached statistical significance.

Table 9.3 shows the *methods* used in suicide attempts differentiated into violent and non-violent methods. In defining violent suicidal behaviour, the suggestions of van Heeringen (van Heeringen *et al.*, 2000) were adopted, counting self-poisoning with drugs or single wrist cuts as non-violent, and other self-inflicted injuries as violent methods. Examples of violent methods in this sample are jumping from

Table 9.3. Methods of suicide attempts

	ATPD n (%)	PS n (%)	BSAD n (%)	Statistical analysis[d]
Number of suicide attempts in whole course of illness	$n = 33^a$	$n = 30^a$	$n = 52^a$	
Non-violent methods[b]	26 (78.8)	21 (70.0)	35 (67.3)	n.s.
Violent methods[c]	7 (21.2)	9 (30.0)	17 (32.7)	n.s.
Number of suicide attempts in acute episode	$n = 11$	$n = 0$	$n = 6$	
Non-violent methods[b]	7 (63.6)	0	2 (33.3)	n.s.
Violent methods[c]	4 (36.4)	0	4 (66.7)	n.s.

[a] Numbers in this table refer to suicide attempts, not subjects.
[b] Drug intoxication, single wrist cuts.
[c] Jumping from a height, gas poisoning, hanging.
[d] No significant differences in pairwise comparisons with χ^2 test or Fisher's exact test.

heights or gas poisoning. When looking at the whole course of the illness, non-violent methods like self-poisoning with drugs or single wrist cuts were most frequent in all groups. During an acute episode of ATPD or of BSAD, violent methods were used somewhat more frequently (Table 9.3). No differences between the diagnostic groups in the method of suicide emerged. To answer the question as to whether the *course of the illness* differed between patients with and without suicidal behaviour, ATPD and control samples were divided into two groups: those with suicidal behaviour during the entire course of the illness and those without. Table 9.4 shows that there are few differences in course parameters between suicidal and non-suicidal patients. In all three clinical groups, patients with suicidal behaviour tended to be younger at the first manifestation of illness than those without. The difference was greatest in patients with Positive Schizophrenia, but still did not reach statistical significance. In patients with Positive Schizophrenia, there was also an association of suicidal behaviour with a higher number of episodes; this association was statistically significant only on trend level. Thus, PS seems to be most closely linked to a longer duration of illness and a higher number of episodes. While this finding should only be interpreted with reservation due to the large number of statistical comparisons calculated, it would be consistent with an association of suicidal behaviour and chronicity in schizophrenia. Also, patients with and without suicidal behaviour during the whole course of illness were compared with regard to outcome parameters. T-tests were calculated to evaluate differences in GAS, WHO/DAS and WHO/PIRS at the first follow-up, and GAS, WHO/DAS and PANSS scores at the end of the prospective follow-up period according to the

Table 9.4. Suicidal behaviour and course features

	ATPD $n = 42$		PS $n = 42$		BSAD $n = 42$	
	n	Mean $\pm$ SD	n	Mean $\pm$ SD	n	Mean $\pm$ SD
Age at first episode (years)						
With suicidal behaviour	15	34.9 $\pm$ 9.1	17	30.4 $\pm$ 10.3[b]	24	27.9 $\pm$ 9.8
Without suicidal behaviour	27	36.2 $\pm$ 12.2	25	38.6 $\pm$ 15.2	18	29.6 $\pm$ 12.2
Length of illness (years)[a]						
With suicidal behaviour	15	10.6 $\pm$ 6.9	16	13.3 $\pm$ 6.9	21	16.2 $\pm$ 8.6
Without suicidal behaviour	24	10.6 $\pm$ 8.7	22	9.4 $\pm$ 7.4	16	20.3 $\pm$ 10.3
Number of episodes[a]						
With suicidal behaviour	15	3.9 $\pm$ 2.1	16	5.6 $\pm$ 3.4[b]	21	8.0 $\pm$ 4.9
Without suicidal behaviour	24	4.6 $\pm$ 4.2	22	3.8 $\pm$ 2.4	16	8.4 $\pm$ 4.1
Annual frequency of episodes[a]						
With suicidal behaviour	15	0.49 $\pm$ 0.31	16	0.49 $\pm$ 0.37	21	0.52 $\pm$ 0.29
Without suicidal behaviour	23	0.51 $\pm$ 0.32	22	0.53 $\pm$ 0.45	16	0.44 $\pm$ 0.20

[a] For calculation of course parameters only patients with completed follow-up were included.
[b] Difference between patients with and without suicidal behaviour in t-test significant on trend level only ($P < 0.10$); all other comparisons not significant.

presence or absence of suicidal behaviour. No differences were found in any of the outcome parameters between patients with and without suicidal behaviour within each diagnostic group. Even after all three groups were combined and the tests were repeated, no differences were found.

In the HASBAP, a substantial rate of suicidal behaviour was found in all psychiatric groups during the whole course of the disorder concerning up to 57% of patients. In 35.7% of ATPD patients, suicidal behaviour was registered at least once during the course, which is comparable to the rate of 40.5% in patients with PS. In the literature, rates of suicide attempts in schizophrenia vary between 20 and 40% (Marneros *et al.*, 1991b; Amador *et al.*, 1996; Gupta *et al.*, 1998; Radomsky *et al.*, 1999), and in schizoaffective psychoses they were found to be around 36.6% (Marneros *et al.*, 1991b) concerning the whole course of the illness. The fact that rates of suicidal behaviour in the sample of the HASBAP range at the higher end of figures reported in the literature can partially be explained by the high proportion of female subjects in this study sample (78.6%), which is characteristic for patients with ATPD (Marneros *et al.*, 2000, 2002a, 2003; Pillmann *et al.*, 2001). Women, in general, are two to three times more likely to attempt suicide than men, whereas, in men, the rate of suicide is two to three times higher (Buda and Tsuang, 1990; Goodwin and Jamison, 1990). While rates of suicidal behaviour in ATPD did not differ significantly from those in PS, rates in BSAD were significantly higher. This might be due to the earlier onset of BSAD compared to ATPD and PS. However, in BSAD subjects, no association was found between presence of suicidal behaviour and length of illness or number of episodes. It has been shown that schizoaffective patients are at an increased risk of suicidal behaviour (mainly during schizodepressive episodes) compared to schizophrenic and affective patients (Marneros *et al.*, 1991b; Radomsky *et al.*, 1999). Some authors assumed that bipolarity further adds to the risk of suicidal behaviour (Bottlender *et al.*, 2000).

Committed suicides followed the same distribution between the diagnostic groups as suicide attempts. There was no committed suicide in ATPD, but two in PS (4.8%) and three in BSAD (7.1%). Suicide rates reported in intermediate and long-term follow-up studies range from about 10 to 15% for schizophrenia (Tsuang, 1978; Drake *et al.*, 1985; Amador *et al.*, 1996; Stephens *et al.*, 1997; Wiersma *et al.*, 1998; Tsuang *et al.*, 1999) and about 19% for schizoaffective psychoses (Angst *et al.*, 1990). Comparing the data of the HASBAP with these rates one has to take into consideration that due to the study design, the period of risk (prospectively observed) was on average 5 years. While suicide attempts could be evaluated over the whole course of the illness, successful suicides could only be registered in the period between index episode and the end of the prospective follow-up. With this limitation in mind, observed suicides are within the expected range for Positive Schizophrenia and Bipolar Schizoaffective Disorder. The absence of completed suicides in ATPD during the observation period could indicate a lower risk of suicide in this group. However, since sample size and prospective follow-up time are still limited, no definite conclusions should be drawn at this time.

Suicide attempts in ATPD mainly occurred during the acute episode. In the ATPD group, the frequency of suicidal behaviour during the acute episode was by far the highest in the investigated samples. This finding may be better understood by taking into account the typical psychopathological features of ATPD: episodes of ATPD are acute and dramatic with a sudden onset, often combined with overwhelming anxiety and agitation (Marneros *et al.*, 2002a, 2003; Pillmann *et al.*, 2001). Thus, suicidal behaviour in ATPD can be expected to occur mainly at the climax of the acute and dramatic psychotic syndrome. This could explain the fact that most suicide attempts in ATPD occurred shortly before admission. In contrast, in schizophrenia, an association was seen between suicidal behaviour and indicators of chronicity (length of illness and number of episodes). Course and outcome features showed no significant association with suicidal behaviour in ATPD patients.

Conclusion: The acute psychotic symptomatology seems to be the main factor influencing suicidal behaviour in Acute and Transient Psychotic Disorder patients, therefore it is more frequent during the acute episode.

10

Comorbidity and somatic findings

ATPD, by definition, are functional psychoses. A diagnosis of an organic psychosis or any other kind of organic mental disorder is not compatible with ATPD. Nevertheless, an 'organic impression' of the symptomatology is not uncommon in ATPD, and may include features such as confusion or disorientation (Murai *et al.*, 1996). A number of authors have suggested that metabolic, endocrinological or epileptic mechanisms play a role in the pathogenesis of Brief and Acute Psychoses (Kleist, 1953; Monroe, 1959; Kurosawa, 1961; Fekkes *et al.*, 1994; Hatotani, 1996). Investigations carried out in India identified antecedent fever as a risk factor for the occurrence of Acute Brief Psychosis (Collins *et al.*, 1996, 1999; Malhotra *et al.*, 1998). In order to investigate the role of somatic illness in ATPD, somatic diagnoses and paraclinical findings in ATPD are reported and compared to PS and ATPD.

Somatic comorbidity

Somatic comorbidity in the three diagnostic groups is reported in Table 10.1. This includes all somatic diagnoses that were documented during the acute episode or elicited in the sociobiographic interview, irrespective of a possible aetiological link to the psychiatric disorder. There was no significant difference between the three diagnostic groups in somatic comorbidity. The diagnoses covered the whole spectrum of medicine and different degrees of severity. In Table 10.2, the prevalence of diagnoses in diagnostic categories of particular relevance is reported (neurological, endocrinological and cardiovascular). No particular pattern of comorbid diagnoses was observed. None of the disorders could be clearly established as an aetiological factor for the psychiatric condition. One female patient with PS suffered from active syphilis infection, but no cerebral involvement was found. The same patient shortly afterwards was diagnosed with chronic myeloid leukaemia. Disorders not listed in Table 10.2 include a wide array of orthopaedic, ophthalmologic, oto-rhino-laryngological and gynaecological diseases.

Table 10.1. Patients with at least one comorbid somatic diagnosis

	ATPD $n = 42$	PS $n = 42$	BSAD $n = 42$	Statistical analysis[a]
Any co-morbid somatic disorder	15 (35.7)	11 (26.2)	14 (33.3)	n.s.
No co-morbid somatic disorder	27 (64.3)	31 (73.8)	28 (66.7)	

[a] No significant differences in pairwise χ^2 tests.

Table 10.2. Somatic diagnoses according to selected diagnostic groups

	ATPD $n = 42$	PS $n = 42$	BSAD $n = 42$
	n (%)	n (%)	n (%)
Neurological diseases (Chapter G of ICD-10)	2 (4.8) Chronic headache Incomplete paraplegia[a]	1 (2.4) Cerebral palsy	0
Endocrinological disease (Chapter E of ICD-10)	3 (7.1) Diabetes mellitus (2x) Goitre	3 (7.1) Diabetes Vitamin-B12-Deficiency Albinism	5 (11.9) Goitre (3x) Diabetes mellitus (2x)
Cardiovascular (Chapter I of ICD-10)	1 (2.4) Hypertension	1 (2.4) Hypertension	1 (2.4) Hypertension
Other severe medical disorders		1 (2.4) Chronic myeloid leukemia and active syphilis (without cerebral involvment)	

No significant differences in pairwise χ^2 tests or Fisher's exact test.
[a] As a result from a suicide attempt (jumped out of a window).

> **Conclusion:** No particular pattern of somatic comorbidity for Acute and Transient Psychotic Disorders can be found. Studies from developing countries that find increased rates of somatic disease in patients with Acute and Transient Psychotic Disorders cannot be confirmed in European samples.

Table 10.3. Abnormal laboratory findings

	ATPD $n = 42$	PS $n = 42$	BSAD $n = 42$	Statistical analysis[a]
Lowered level of B12	1 (2.4)	2 (4.8)	1 (2.4)	n.s.
Thyroid abnormalities[b]	4 (9.5)	2 (4.8)	3 (7.1)	n.s.

[a] No significant differences in pairwise comparisons with Fisher's exact test.
[b] Slightly lowered or elevated levels of peripheral hormones or TSH, below the threshold of a clinical diagnosis of thyroid dysfunction.

Laboratory findings

Among the laboratory investigations performed routinely in every patient, two parameters are of particular importance because they could possibly be pathogenetically connected to the development of ATPD: thyroid hormones (T3, T4, TSH) and vitamin B12 (Mall, 1952; Kurosawa, 1961). Both parameters belonged to the routine work-up during the period of investigation. Table 10.3 gives the number of patients in whom abnormalities of these parameters were observed. In only one patient with PS was the lowered level of B12 of clinical significance (see Table 10.2). In all other cases, the laboratory abnormalities were below the threshold of a clinical diagnosis.

> Conclusion: In Acute and Transient Psychotic Disorders, there is no indication of an increased prevalence of somatic disorders in general, or of any specific somatic diagnosis when compared to Positive Schizophrenia and Bipolar Schizoaffective Disorders. In comparison to the clinical control groups, in Acute and Transient Psychotic Disorders no elevated rates of (subclinical) abnormalities of thyroid function or vitamin B12 could be observed.

Neuroradiological findings

Cerebral atrophy has long been described as a feature of schizophrenic psychoses (Huber, 1957) and has been corroborated by numerous studies with cerebral computed tomography (CCT) and nuclear resonance tomography (NMR) (overview in Shenton et al., 2001). For atypical psychoses, a lower rate of cerebral atrophy as determined by CCT was found in comparison to schizophrenia. This finding was supported by a study on cycloid psychoses conducted by Höffler and co-workers (1997).

Interestingly, not all researchers who investigated cycloid psychoses found *lower* rates of cerebral atrophy in comparison to schizophrenia. In particular, the Beckmann group in Würzburg favours the hypothesis that cycloid psychoses are

Table 10.4. Radiological findings in the three diagnostic groups[a]

	ATPD n = 39	PS n = 35	BSAD n = 31	
	n (%)	n (%)	n (%)	Statistical analysis[b]
Normal	28 (71.8)	27 (77.1)	20 (64.5)	n.s.
Ischemia	1 (2.6)	1 (2.9)	0	n.s.
Atrophy	7 (17.9)	5 (14.3)	10 (32.3)	n.s.
Other[c]	3 (7.7)	2 (5.7)	1 (3.2)	n.s.

[a] 99 patients with cranial computed tomography, 3 with nuclear magnetic resonance tomography
[b] No significant differences in pairwise comparisons with χ^2 test or Fisher's exact test.
[c] Findings of questionable pathological valence (calcifications, small suspected hypodensities).

distinguished by *higher* rates of exogenous disturbances during pregnancy and childbirth than other forms of endogenous psychoses (Stöber *et al.*, 1997). The rationale for this argument has been described on page 33 and need not be repeated here. In fact, Franzek and co-workers (1996) found evidence in favour of an increased rate of CCT abnormalities in cycloid psychoses.

In the HASBAP, there was an attempt to determine whether abnormalities of the brain scans differentiate between ATPD and the clinical control groups. As part of the standard diagnostic work-up, a computed tomography of the head was performed in most patients. In some patients ($n = 3$), a nuclear resonance tomography of the head was also performed. All CT and NMR scans were reviewed by certified radiologists. Table 10.4 gives the results of these examinations. It is shown that, for most patients, no pathological findings were recorded. If there were any abnormalities, these mostly consisted of signs of atrophy. For the subsample with cerebral atrophy, the localisation of the atrophy is reported in Table 10.5. The most frequent localisation was frontal in all groups investigated. There was no specific pattern of atrophy that distinguished ATPD from the other clinical groups.

In a third analysis, 30 CCT examinations of patients with ATPD and 29 CCT examinations of patients with PS (all those available for this analysis) were investigated by independent raters using the CT Rating Scale for Schizophrenia (Smith *et al.*, 1997). This instrument allows the rating of routine CT scans to be assessed in nine regions (Sylvian Fissure, temporal lobe sulci, frontal sulci, medial-frontal sulci, lateral and parietal-occipital sulci, third ventricle, and the body, frontal horns, and temporal horns of the lateral ventricles). Each of the nine ratings is made using a seven-point scale with photographs of each brain region used as anchor points for ratings of 1, 3, 5 and 7. This standardised method of visual assessment is robust and the use of unstandardised scanning procedures and more than one

Table 10.5. Localisation of cerebral atrophy in CCT or NMR in the three diagnostic groups[a]

	ATPD $n = 7$	PS $n = 5$	BSAD $n = 10$	
	n (%)	n (%)	n (%)	Statistical analysis[a]
Frontal	3 (43)	3 (60)	5 (50)	n.s.
Temporal	0	1 (20)	2 (20)	n.s.
Cerebellum	2 (29)	0	3 (30)	n.s.
Generalised	2 (29)	1 (20)	0	n.s.

[a] No significant differences in pairwise comparisons with Fisher's exact test.

Table 10.6. Cerebral atrophy indices (CT Rating Scale for Schizophrenia) in ATPD and PS

	ATPD $n = 30$	PS $n = 29$	
	Mean ± SD	Mean ± SD	Statistical analysis[a]
Cortical atrophy index	16.3 ± 7.3	18.5 ± 7.2	n.s.
Ventricular atrophy index	13.6 ± 7.1	14.1 ± 6.2	n.s.
Sum score	29.9 ± 13.3	32.6 ± 12.0	n.s.

[a] No significant differences in pairwise t-tests.

scanner has minimal influence on ratings (Smith *et al.*, 1997). Raters were blind to patient data including diagnosis and age. Prior to the ratings, the inter-rater reliability has been determined and found to be >0.80 for all measures (intra-class correlation coefficient). Scores for the different regions were added up to generate an index of cortical atrophy, an index of ventricular atrophy and a sum score. Table 10.6 gives the scores for ATPD and PS patients in comparison. No significant differences were found. There was a strong correlation with age, in particular for the cortical atrophy index, but also for the ventricular atrophy index and the sum score.

Conclusion: The data from the Halle Study on Brief and Acute Psychoses do not show any significant difference in CCT and NMR cerebral diagnostic between Acute and Transient Psychotic Disorders and the clinical control groups. In particular, Acute and Transient Psychotic Disorder and Positive Schizophrenia patients show signs of atrophy in the same rates. Thus, neither the hypothesis of a lowered prevalence of CCT abnormalities, nor the hypothesis (as discussed above) that CCT abnormalities in Acute and Transient Psychotic Disorders should be elevated, can be supported.

EEG findings

The EEG findings of the HASBAP are presented and discussed extensively for two reasons. Firstly, the HASBAP was the first study reporting EEG data on ATPD. Secondly, as already pointed out (p. 29), some authors assumed that the so-called 'atypical psychosis' of Japanese psychiatry (which is partially a synonym for ATPD) has some relationships to epilepsy. Mitsuda (1965) and Hatotani (1996) supposed 'atypical psychosis' to be nosologically positioned between schizophrenia, affective psychosis and epilepsy. A close association between epilepsy and psychopathological syndromes characterised by acute onset, polymorphic symptomatology and good prognosis is also presumed by other authors (Monroe, 1959; Tucker *et al.*, 1986). Recently, Inui and co-workers (1998) reported further evidence of this association.

To investigate the question of electroencephalographic abnormalities in ATPD, EEG recordings of all three patient groups were analysed (Röttig, 2001). From the total of 126 patients, 119 underwent an electroencephalographic examination. The remaining 7 patients refused the EEG examination. The EEG examinations were performed for at least 15 min, including provocation for 3 min by hyperventilation. Electrode placement followed the international 10/20 system. The evaluation was done visually using a coding scheme already employed in a previous study (Pillmann *et al.*, 2000b). Abnormalities were classified as slowing of the dominant occipital rhythm, epileptiform activity as defined below, focal abnormalities and diffuse or intermittent slowing. For each item, ordinal scores were used with four categories as a rule (absent, slight, medium, severe abnormality). For epileptiform activity, borderline findings were differentiated from unambiguous epileptiform discharges (spikes, multiple spikes or spike-wave complexes). The inter-rater reliability was demonstrated to be satisfactory (Pillmann *et al.*, 2000b). All EEGs were evaluated with the investigator being blind to the subject and group assignment.

Medication status at the time of the EEG examination was recorded. The different medications were grouped into categories with a similar effect on the EEG (see Table 10.7) according to the proposal of Saletu (Saletu *et al.*, 1987; Saletu, 1992). Two further groups not originally considered by Saletu (1992) were added (carbamazepine and lithium). Table 10.8 reports the EEG findings in the three psychotic groups. In none of the patients were epileptiform discharges found before hyperventilation (Table 10.8). Non-specific signs of increased cerebral excitability were found in three patients with ATPD, two patients with Positive Schizophrenia and one patient with Bipolar Schizoaffective Disorder. One PS patient showed spike-wave complexes after hyperventilation. The differences between the diagnostic groups were not statistically significant. Similarly, no statistically significant differences between ATPD, PS and BSAD were found with regard to the presence of localised dysfunction or diffuse slowing.

Table 10.7. Medication groups for EEG investigation

1. Low-potency antipsychotics
2. High-potency antipsychotics
3. Thymoleptic antidepressants
4. Thymeretic antidepressants
5. Tranquillisers
6. Lithium[a]
7. Carbamazepine[a]

[a] Not considered by the used proposal.

Table 10.8. Relationship between diagnostic groups and EEG parameters

	ATPD $n = 39$	PS $n = 40$	BSAD $n = 40$	
	n (%)	n (%)	n (%)	Statistical analysis[a]
Increased cerebral excitability				
None	36 (92.3%)	37 (92.5%)	39 (97.5%)	n.s.
Borderline findings	3 (7.7%)	2 (5.0%)	1 (2.5%)	n.s.
Epileptiform discharges only after hyperventilation	0 (0%)	1 (2.5%)	0 (0%)	n.s.
Epileptiform discharges before hyperventilation	0 (0%)	0 (0%)	0 (0%)	n.s.
Intermittent slowing				
None	28 (71.8%)	29 (72.5%)	18 (45.0%)	BSAD < PS* BSAD < ATPD*
Light	2 (5.1%)	5 (12.5%)	9 (22.5%)	BSAD > ATPD*
Medium	7 (17.9%)	4 (10.0%)	12 (30.0%)	BSAD > PS*
Severe	2 (5.1%)	2 (5.0%)	1 (2.5%)	n.s.
Diffuse slowing				
None	39 (100%)	40 (100%)	38 (95%)	n.s.
Light	0 (0%)	0 (0%)	2 (5%)	n.s.
Medium	0 (0%)	0 (0%)	0 (0%)	n.s.
Severe	0 (0%)	0 (0%)	0 (0%)	n.s.

[a] Only pairwise comparisons with significant differences (χ^2 test or Fisher's exact test, two-tailed) are shown.
* $P < 0.05$, n.s. no significance.

Intermittent slowing was found significantly more often in the BSAD patient group than in ATPD and PS (Table 10.8). This abnormality was displayed by 11 (18.2%) patients with ATPD, 11 (17.5%) with PS, and 22 (55%) with BSAD. However, this difference might have been confounded by the influence of psychopharmacological medication. To evaluate this possibility, in a first step the association between the EEG parameter 'intermittent slowing' and the above-mentioned medication groups was investigated. In univariate comparisons, a significant relationship was found between 'intermittent slowing' and a medication with 'high-potency antipsychotics' ($P = 0.020$) and 'low-potency antipsychotics' ($P = 0.017$), as well as with lithium ($P = 0.048$). In a second step, an analysis of variance was performed (ANOVA) with 'intermittent slowing' as the independent variable to investigate the relative effects of the factors 'diagnostic group' and medication. The three groups of medication shown to be associated with intermittent slowing along with diagnosis were entered as independent variables. The only significant main effect was for 'low-potency antipsychotics' ($F = 3.967$, $P = 0.049$), whereas the factors 'diagnostic group' ($F = 1.819$, $P = 0.167$), lithium ($F = 1.275$, $P = 0.261$) and 'high-potency antipsychotics' ($F = 0.944$, $P = 0.333$) proved to be of no significant effect. It can be concluded that the higher prevalence of intermittent slowing in BSAD patients is not a characteristic of this diagnostic group, but rather a consequence of the frequency of low-potency antipsychotics in this group.

Summary and conclusions from EEG findings

To our knowledge, the HASBAP was the first to report EEG findings in ATPD (F23, ICD-10). Some earlier studies investigated EEG findings in patients with syndromes similar to ATPD (Monroe, 1959; Tucker *et al.*, 1986; Hatotani, 1996; Inui *et al.*, 1998). In contrast to these studies, no evidence was found of increased cerebral excitability in ATPD compared with positive schizophrenic and bipolar schizoaffective controls. Also, with regard to other investigated EEG parameters, no differences between ATPD and controls were found.

The failure of the HASBAP to confirm the findings of the mentioned authors may be accounted for by several factors, including differences in sample selection and use of different methods to elicit epileptiform activity. It must be noted that only one of the cited studies (Inui *et al.*, 1998) used operational criteria for diagnosis (DSM-IV), and none of the studies explicitly investigated ATPD according to ICD-10. In the Monroe study (1959), a small and selected sample was used without controls. Tucker and co-workers (1986) investigated a highly selected sample of 20 psychotic patients, but no controls. The patients had symptoms similar to ATPD, but following more recent diagnostic criteria, most of the conditions would be classified as epileptic psychoses.

Monroe (1959) used a drug activation method with alpha-chloralose, which is rarely used today (Niedermeyer and Lopez da Silva, 1993). A high rate of alpha-chloralose-induced EEG abnormalities was also found in other diagnostic groups by Monroe and Mickle (1967). Therefore, this might be an unspecific phenomenon.

Hatotani (1996) reported a lower threshold for spike-wave complexes following administration of epileptogenic drugs in atypical psychosis, a concept similar to that of ATPD.

In the HASBAP, hyperventilation was used as a method of provocation, but no epileptogenic drugs were used to provoke epileptiform activity. The possibility cannot be excluded that, in the HASBAP sample, the use of such a procedure would have led to differences between diagnostic groups. However, as mentioned above, the method of drug activation is controversial and rarely used today because of its low specificity and doubtful validity, as well as for ethical considerations (Niedermeyer and Lopez da Silva, 1993).

> Conclusion: The EEG findings, but also the clinical symptomatology and course, do not support the assumption of epileptic patterns in Acute and Transient Psychotic Disorders. Moreover, no specific EEG pattern can be found in any of the three psychotic groups.

Part III

Issues of nosology

11

Defining the brief, acute and transient psychotic disorders: the polymorphic psychotic core

The boundaries of homogeneity

Both APA and WHO try to define 'Brief Psychoses' and '*Acute and Transient Psychotic Disorder*', respectively, by using the time factor (duration of an episode of the disturbance is at least 1 day, but less than 1 month) as well as the cultural aspect (a symptom is not included if it is a culturally sanctioned response pattern, see p. 7) and by the exclusion of the effects of a substance or of general medical conditions. The WHO tries to achieve homogeneity on the one hand by using similar exclusion criteria like those of DSM-IV (time factor, organic cause, etc.), but on the other by defining subgroups (see p. 7ff). The first way, the time factor, however, applied by the WHO is somewhat more complicated than that of the APA. The first time factor used by the WHO concerns the development of symptoms (the time-interval between the first appearance of any psychotic symptoms and the presentation of the fully developed disorder should not exceed 2 weeks). And the second factor, the duration of an episode, depends on the type of the subgroup: the total duration of the disorder in the subgroups with schizophrenic symptoms (F23.1: Acute Polymorphic Psychotic Disorders *with* Symptoms of Schizophrenia, F23.2: Acute Schizophrenia-like Psychotic Disorders) must not exceed 1 month. This is also valid for the unspecified type (F23.8). In subcategories without symptoms of schizophrenia (F23.0: Acute Polymorphic Psychotic Disorders *without* Symptoms of Schizophrenia, F23.3: Predominantly Delusional Psychotic Disorder) the duration of the episode may be up to 3 months.

The second way followed by the WHO is the phenomenological approach by defining subgroups mainly based on the presence or absence of first-rank psychotic symptoms:

- Acute Polymorphic Psychotic Disorder *with* Symptoms of Schizophrenia,
- Acute Polymorphic Psychotic Disorders *without* Symptoms of Schizophrenia,
- Schizophrenia-like Psychotic Disorders (with symptoms of schizophrenia),

- Acute Predominantly Delusional Psychotic Disorders (without symptoms of schizophrenia; the group of other and the group of unspecified acute psychotic disorders may or may not have schizophrenic symptoms).

But there is no research on the topic of whether such division of several subgroups is necessary or not.

Considering the finding that there is no difference between the DSM-IV 'Brief Psychoses' and the ICD-10 'Acute and Transient Psychotic Disorders' (Pillmann et al., 2002), as well as the finding that the WHO group is more voluminous, we concentrated our intentions regarding the question of homogeneity of Brief and Acute Psychoses on the WHO group of 'Acute and Transient Psychotic Disorders'.

The definition of ATPD as given by the WHO in ICD-10, their various synonyms and conceptual roots as well as their various subclassifications, can give rise to the assumption that this group is an inhomogeneous group of psychotic disorders. It is indeed possible that some of them do have a stronger relationship to 'typical' schizophrenia and some of them do not. Inhomogeneity cannot be absolutely eliminated, not only for ATPD, but also for all groups of mental disorders, at least as long as we have only a very incomplete knowledge of their aetiology. But, perhaps inhomogeneity can be somewhat limited by using strict definitions and valid criteria!

The problem concerns, however, the question: what are the most valid defining criteria? We think that the most valid criteria for the definition of a mental disorder, especially a psychotic disorder, have to be the same as those defining diseases in general (i.e. signs and symptoms in characteristic connection with biological findings). But, unfortunately, we will need a long time to achieve this diagnostic level in psychiatry. In fact, to achieve this level, it is necessary to define at an earlier stage disorders or groups of disorders using 'soft criteria', such as symptomatological and phenomenological signs without connection to specific biological findings, or 'semi-soft criteria', like gender, age at onset, premorbid features and functional level, course and outcome of a disorder. Specific biological–somatological and genetic findings can be labelled 'hard criteria', which we unfortunately do not have completely or not at all. The WHO obviously had no choice but to apply only 'soft criteria' (i.e. criteria based mainly on the phenomenological approach) in the definition of Acute and Transient Psychotic Disorders (and other disorders), as well as the APA for the Brief Psychoses. The reason for the limited choice was not only the absence of 'hard' defining criteria, but also the lack of systematic research estimating 'semi-soft' criteria (WHO, 1992; Marneros et al., 2000, 2002; Pillmann et al., 2002).

The authors of the WHO classification paid particular attention to the so-called 'schizophrenic first-rank symptoms' (Schneider, 1959; Mellor, 1982; Marneros, 1984). In this sense, the ICD-10 differentiates the 'Acute Polymorphic Psychoses' in 'with' and 'without symptoms of schizophrenia', referring mainly to first-rank symptoms. Similarly, the WHO defines the 'Acute Schizophrenia-like Disorders' by the presence of schizophrenic symptoms (first-rank symptoms) and by the absence of polymorphic symptomatology (WHO, 1993) (see p. 11).

The distinction of psychotic disorders simply and alone according to the presence or absence of schizophrenic first-rank symptoms is no longer valid: schizophrenic first-rank symptoms are not a *conditio sine qua non* for the diagnosis of schizophrenia because they are not always present (Koehler, 1983; Marneros, 1984; Marneros *et al.*, 1987). They can be found in schizoaffective disorders (see contributions in Marneros and Tsuang, 1986, 1990; and Marneros *et al.*, 1991b), as well as in organic psychotic disorders (Schneider, 1959; Marneros, 1988). According to DSM-IV, they can also be present in affective psychotic disorders, a position, however, which is very problematic. But, nevertheless, the result is that obviously schizophrenic first-rank symptoms are not specific.

To examine the question of whether the differentiation of ATPD in their groups is valid and necessary, statistical investigations comparing all available data were carried out as follows:

- Comparison of 'Acute Polymorphic Psychotic Disorder *With* Symptoms of Schizophrenia' (ICD-10 F23.0) versus '*Without* Symptoms of Schizophrenia' (ICD-10 F23.1)
- Comparison of 'Acute Polymorphic Psychotic Disorders' (ICD-10 F23.0 and F23.1) vs. 'Acute Schizophrenia-like Psychotic Disorder' (ICD-10 F23.2)
- Comparison of 'Acute Polymorphic Psychotic Disorders' vs. the other clinical control groups of the HASBAP (Positive Schizophrenia, Bipolar Schizoaffective Disorder).

The comparisons concerned the domains showed on Table 11.1. The question was whether there is any necessity to distinguish the Acute Polymorphic Psychotic Disorders into two groups based on the presence of schizophrenic symptoms. The summary of the findings concerning the comparison between the two groups is given in Tables 11.2, 11.3 and 11.4. *No significant differences between the Polymorphic Psychotic Disorders with or without schizophrenic symptoms were found.* The small number of patients belonging to the two groups is a major limitation for the statistical analysis. That is, however, not a weakness of the HASBAP, but a diagnosis-dependent limitation: patients having the above diagnosis are relatively rare not only among clinical subjects but also in general, at least in the industrialised world. Nevertheless, the above findings support findings of other studies that the so-called 'schizophrenic symptoms' (i.e. 'first-rank symptoms') are not specific and do not have a diagnostic or predictive validity (Koehler, 1983; Marneros, 1984, 1988; Marneros *et al.*, 1991b; Carpenter *et al.*, 1995). As already mentioned, it is well known that first-rank symptoms according to Schneider (Schneider, 1950, 1959) (e.g. delusional perceptions, thought withdrawal, thought broadcasting, thought insertion, thought hearing and the psychotic experience of being influenced) can also be found in other disorders

Table 11.1. Domains compared in the subgroup comparisons

Sociobiographical data
Family data
Premorbid personality
Gender
Age at onset
Kind of onset
Life events
Development of the symptomatology
Duration of the psychotic period
Suicidal behaviour
Treatment parameters
Somatological findings
Course
Outcome

besides schizophrenia as already mentioned (for example, schizoaffective, epileptic, and chronic-organic psychoses, or after intoxication, Marneros, 1988). Additionally, not all schizophrenic patients have schizophrenic first-rank symptoms during the episode: during the first episodes, only a minority of patients have first-rank symptoms and only during the long-term course do more and more schizophrenic patients show such symptoms (Mellor et al., 1981; Mellor, 1982; Koehler, 1983; Marneros, 1988). *In other words, the presence or absence of first-rank schizophrenic symptoms cannot distinguish the Acute Polymorphic Disorders into subgroups. Obviously, the polymorphism of the symptomatology has a much more discriminating power than the presence of first-rank schizophrenic symptoms.* This provides clear support for the opinions of the creators of the concept of cycloid disorders (Kleist, 1924; Leonhard, 1957; Perris, 1974; Perris and Brockington, 1981; Sigmund and Mundt, 1999; Beckmann and Franzek, 2001) as well as that of the bouffée délirante (Magnan and Legrain, 1895; Pull et al., 1983; Pichot, 1986a).

Conclusion: The WHO distinction of 'Acute Polymorphic Disorder' into the two categories 'with' and 'without schizophrenic symptoms' cannot be supported. Such a distinction is unwarranted and is therefore unnecessary. Not schizophrenic first rank symptoms, but the symptomatologic polymorphism carries the most relevant distinguishing power. We suggest that the ICD-10 subtype F23.0 ('with' schizophrenic symptoms) and F23.1 ('without' schizophrenic symptoms) be put together.

Table 11.2. Comparison between Acute Polymorphic Psychotic Disorders With and Without Symptoms of Schizophrenia (part 1)

	Acute Polymorphic Psychotic Disorder without Symptoms of Schizophrenia F23.0 $n = 14$	Acute Polymorphic Psychotic Disorder with Symptoms of Schizophrenia F23.1 $n = 14$	P
	n (%)	n (%)	
Female gender	10 (71.4)	13 (92.9)	0.326[c]
Broken home	5 (35.7)	9 (64.3)	0.131[a]
Disturbance of early development			0.368[a]
No disturbance	13 (92.9)	13 (92.9)	
Suspected disturbance	1 (7.1)	0	
Definite disturbance	0	1 (7.1)	
Obstetric complications			0.222[a]
No complication reported	11 (78.6)	14 (100.0)	
Complications suspected	3 (21.4)	0	
Definite complications	0	0	
Level of education			0.320[b]
Very low	3 (21.4)	1 (7.1)	
Low	2 (14.3)	5 (35.7)	
Medium	4 (28.6)	8 (57.1)	
High	5 (35.7)	0	
First-degree relatives			
Any psychiatric disorder	6 (42.9)	5 (35.7)	0.699[a]
Major psychotic or affective disorder	4 (28.6)	1 (7.1)	0.326[c]
Alcohol abuse	0	1 (7.1)	1.0[c]
Premorbid personality			0.916[a]
Obsessoid	3 (21.4)	3 (21.4)	
Sthenic/high self-confidence	3 (21.4)	2 (14.3)	
Asthenic/low self-confidence	5 (35.7)	6 (42.9)	
Nervous-tense	2 (14.3)	1 (7.1)	
Undeterminable	1 (7.1)	2 (14.3)	

Values given as Mean ± SD or n (%).

[a] χ^2 test.

[b] Mann–Whitney U-test.

[c] Fisher's exact test, two-tailed.

Table 11.3. Comparison between Acute Polymorphic Psychotic Disorder With and Without Symptoms of Schizophrenia (part 2)

	Acute Polymorphic Psychotic Disorder without Symptoms of Schizophrenia F23.0	Acute Polymorphic Psychotic Disorder without Symptoms of Schizophrenia F23.1	
	$n = 14$	$n = 14$	P
Social interactions before onset			0.373^a
Many contacts	8 (57.1)	11 (78.6)	
Few contacts	5 (35.7)	3 (21.4)	
Socially withdrawn	1 (7.1)	0	
Heterosexual relationship before onset	13 (92.9)	14 (100)	1.0^d
Employed at onset	10 (71.4)	10 (71.4)	1.0^d
Age at onset	33.8 ± 8.1	35.9 ± 7.7	0.498^b
Age at index episode	42.0 ± 12.5	42.3 ± 10.0	0.949^b
Number of episodes before index	2.5 ± 4.3	1.7 ± 2.5	0.562^b
Index episode is first episode	6 (42.9)	6 (42.9)	1.0^a
Duration of psychotic period	12.0 ± 8.6	22.1 ± 17.8	0.066^b
Duration of inpatient treatment	36.4 ± 26.8	33.9 ± 20.8	0.791^b
Mode of onset of the acute episode			1.0^c
Abrupt	7 (50)	7 (50)	
Acute	7 (50)	7 (50)	
Subacute/chronic	0	0	
Features of the acute episode			
With acute stress	1 (7.1)	3 (21.4)	0.596^d
Life event before onset	4 (28.6)	8 (57.1)	0.127^a
Continuity of pharmacotherapy at discharge	13 (92.9)	13 (92.9)	1.0^d
Atrophy in cranial CT	2 (14.3)	3 (21.4)	1.0^d
Suicidal thoughts/suicide attempts during the acute episode	4 (28.6)	2 (14.3)	0.648^d

Values given as Mean ± s.d. or n (%). For some items slightly reduced n due to unclear cases.

[a] χ^2 test.

[b] t-test, two-tailed.

[c] Mann–Whitney U-test.

[d] Fisher's exact test, two-tailed.

Table 11.4. Comparison between Acute Polymorphic Psychotic Disorder With and Without Symptoms of Schizophrenia (part 3)

	Acute Polymorphic Psychotic Disorder with Symptoms of Schizophrenia F23.0	Acute Polymorphic Psychotic Disorder without Symptoms of Schizophrenia F23.1	
	$n = 12$	$n = 13$	P
Relapse until end of prospective follow-up	9 (62.2)	12 (92.3)	0.322[a]
Number of relapses/year until end of prospective follow-up	0.34 ± 0.29	0.39 ± 0.32	0.684[b]
GAS score at the end of the prospective follow-up period	85.9 ± 6.3	84.6 ± 10.9	0.721[b]
DAS global score at the end of the prospective follow-up period	0.33 ± 0.49	0.38 ± 0.77	0.846[b]
PANSS scores at the end of the prospective follow-up period			
Positive symptoms	7.0 ± 0.0	7.7 ± 1.4	0.109[b]
Negative symptoms	9.2 ± 4.11	9.5 ± 5.0	0.842[b]
General symptoms	17.4 ± 1.6	18.4 ± 2.5	0.258[b]
Persisting alterations at the end of the prospective follow-up period	3 (25.0)	2 (15.4)	0.645[b]
Psychosocial status at the end of the prospective follow-up period			
Disability Pension	5 (41.7)	5 (38.5)	1.0[a]
Stable heterosexual relationship	9 (75.0)	10 (76.9)	1.0[a]
Full autarky	11 (91.7)	12 (92.3)	1.0[a]
Pharmacotherapy at follow-up	7 (58.3)	10 (76.9)	0.411[a]
Suicide attempts during whole course of illness	3 (25.0)	5 (38.5)	0.673[a]

Values given as Mean ± SD or n (%).

[a] Fisher's exact test, two-tailed.

[b] t-test, two-tailed.

Is the 'Acute Schizophrenia-like Psychosis' simply schizophrenia?

According to ICD-10, the main difference between 'Acute Schizophrenia-like Disorders' and 'schizophrenia' concerns the criterion 'duration of the symptoms'. Symptoms lasting less than 1 month qualify for a diagnosis of 'Schizophrenia-like Psychotic Disorder', symptoms lasting more than 1 month qualify for a diagnosis of 'schizophrenia'. It is therefore a crucial issue whether this criterion is valid enough to combine the 'Acute Schizophrenia-like Psychoses' with 'Acute Polymorphic

Table 11.5. Comparison between Acute Polymorphic Psychotic Disorder and Acute Schizophrenia-like Psychotic Disorder (part 1)

	Acute Polymorphic Psychotic Disorder F23.0/1 $n = 28$	Acute Schizophrenia-like Psychotic Disorder F23.2 $n = 11$	Statistical analysis[a]
	n (%)	n (%)	P
Female gender	23 (82.1)	7 (63.6)	0.238[c]
Broken home	14 (50.0)	3 (27.3)	0.288[c]
Disturbance of early development			0.661[a]
No disturbance reported	26 (92.9)	11 (100)	
Suspected disturbance	1 (3.6)	0	
Definite disturbance	1 (3.6)	0	
Obstetric complications			0.208[a]
No complication reported	25 (89.3)	8 (72.7)	
Complications suspected	3 (10.7)	2 (18.2)	
Definite complications	0	1 (9.1)	
Level of education			0.557[b]
Very low	4 (14.3)	2 (18.2)	
Low	7 (25.0)	2 (18.2)	
Medium	12 (42.9)	3 (27.3)	
High	5 (17.9)	4 (36.4)	
First-degree relatives			
Any psychiatric disorder	11 (39.3)	2 (18.2)	0.276[c]
Major psychotic or affective disorder	5 (17.9)	1 (9.1)	0.655[c]
Alcohol abuse	1 (3.6)	0	1.0[c]
Premorbid personality			0.344[a]
Obsessoid	6 (21.4)	1 (9.1)	
Sthenic/high self-confident	5 (17.9)	0	
Asthenic/low self-confident	11 (39.3)	8 (72.7)	
Nervous-tense	3 (10.7)	1 (9.1)	
Undeterminable	3 (10.7)	1 (9.1)	

[a] χ^2 test.

[b] Mann–Whitney U-test.

[c] Fisher's exact test, two-tailed.

Psychotic Disorders' within the ATPD. To answer this question, all available data were compared in the same way as between the polymorphic groups. A summary of the findings can be found in Tables 11.5, 11.6 and 11.7. The limitations of a

Table 11.6. Comparison between Acute Polymorphic Psychotic Disorder and Acute Schizophrenia-like Psychotic Disorder (part 2)

	Acute Polymorphic Psychotic Disorder F23.0/1	Acute Schizophrenia-like Psychotic Disorder F23.2	Statistical analysis[a]
	$n = 28$	$n = 11$	P
Social interactions before onset			0.661[b]
Many contacts	19 (67.9)	8 (72.7)	
Few contacts	8 (28.6)	2 (18.2)	
Socially withdrawn	1 (3.6)	1 (9.1)	
Stable heterosexual relationship before onset	27 (96.4)	8 (72.7)	0.060[c]
Employed at first episode	20 (71.4)	5 (45.5)	0.156[c]
Age at onset	34.8 ± 7.9	33.9 ± 13.4	0.783[a]
Age at index episode	42.2 ± 11.1	35.7 ± 13.1	0.130[a]
Number of episodes before index	2.1 ± 3.5	0.27 ± 0.65	0.095[a]
Index episode is first episode	12 (42.9)	9 (81.8)	0.028[b]
Duration of psychotic period	17.1 ± 14.7	18.3 ± 9.8	0.804[a]
Duration of inpatient treatment	35.1 ± 23.5	35.1 ± 27.4	0.995[a]
Mode of onset of the acute episode			0.086[c]
Abrupt	14 (50.0)	2 (18.2)	
Acute	14 (50.0)	9 (81.8)	
Subacute/chronic	0	0	
Features of the acute episode			
With acute stress	4 (14.3)	0	0.309[c]
Life event before onset	12 (42.9)	6 (54.5)	0.510[b]
Continuity of pharmacotherapy at discharge	26 (92.9)	11 (100)	1.0[c]
Atrophy in cranial CT	5 (17.9)	1 (9.1)	0.655[c]
Suicidal thoughts/suicide attempts during acute episode	6 (21.4)	5 (45.5)	0.234[c]

Values given as Mean ± SD or n (%).

[a] t-test, two-tailed.

[b] χ^2 test.

[c] Fisher's exact test, two-tailed.

statistical comparison between the Polymorphic and Schizophrenia-like Acute Psychotic disorders according to the ICD definition are stronger than those of the former comparison, because the group of the Schizophrenia-like Psychotic Disorders in this study is very limited in number. But again it has to be pointed out that this is not a weakness of the HASBAP, but rather is diagnosis dependent. Nevertheless, in spite of this limitation, such a comparison can give some indications for further research.

Table 11.7. Comparison between Acute Polymorphic Psychotic Disorder and Acute Schizophrenia-like Psychotic Disorder (part 3)

	Acute Polymorphic Psychotic Disorder F23.0/1	Acute Schizophrenia-like Psychotic Disorder F23.2	Statistical analysis[a]
	$n = 25$	$n = 11$	
Relapse until end of prospective follow-up	21 (84.0)	8 (72.7)	0.650[b]
Number of relapses/year until end of prospective follow-up	0.37 ± 0.30	0.34 ± 0.38	0.615[a]
Number of relapses	1.68 ± 1.31	1.82 ± 1.66	0.790[a]
GAS score at the end of the prospective follow-up period	85.2 ± 8.8	71.9 ± 22.7	0.015[a]
DAS global score at the end of the prospective follow-up period	0.36 ± 0.64	1.18 ± 1.47	0.024[a]
PANSS scores at the end of the prospective follow-up period			
Positive symptoms	7.4 ± 1.1	9.8 ± 5.6	0.038[a]
Negative symptoms	9.4 ± 4.5	13.6 ± 8.8	0.060[a]
General Symptoms	17.9 ± 2.1	23.5 ± 10.5	0.015[a]
Persisting alterations at the end of the prospective follow-up period	5 (20.0)	6 (54.5)	0.056[b]
Psychosocial status at the end of the prospective follow-up period			
Disability pension	10 (40.0)	4 (36.4)	1.0[b]
Stable heterosexual relationship	19 (76.0)	7 (63.6)	0.454[b]
Full autarky	23 (92.0)	9 (81.8)	0.570[b]
Pharmacotherapy at follow-up	17 (68.0)	9 (81.8)	0.688[b]
Suicide attempts during whole course of illness	8 (32.0)	4 (36.4)	1.0[b]

Values given as mean ± SD or n (%).
[a] t-test, two-tailed.
[b] Fisher's exact test.

The most important finding is that patients with Acute Schizophrenia-like Psychoses show a significantly less favourable outcome than patients with Acute Polymorphic Psychoses in terms of global functioning, disability, positive symptoms, negative symptoms and general symptoms. Patients with Acute Schizophrenia-like Psychoses are therefore more similar to patients with schizophrenia than patients with Acute Polymorphic Psychoses.

> Conclusions: Schizophrenia-like disorders are perhaps closer to schizophrenia. It seems that the category 'Acute and Transient Psychotic Disorder' of the ICD-10 could be much more homogeneous if the 'Acute Polymorphic Psychotic Disorders' are not combined with the 'Acute Schizophrenia-like Psychotic Disorders'.

'Acute Polymorphic Psychotic Disorder' and 'Acute Schizophrenia-like Psychotic Disorder' vs. Positive Schizophrenia and Bipolar Schizoaffective Disorder

The hypothesis was explored of whether the subgroup of ATPD 'Acute Polymorphic Psychotic Disorders', which are very similar to both 'cycloid psychoses' and 'bouffée délirante' (Pillmann et al., 2001; Pillmann and Marneros, 2003), can be distinguished more clearly from the other psychotic groups (Positive Schizophrenia and Bipolar Schizoaffective Disorder) than Acute Schizophrenia-like Psychotic Disorder. For this purpose, the same investigations and the same comparisons were repeated separately for Acute Polymorphic Psychotic Disorders and Acute Schizophrenia-like Psychotic Disorder that were previously carried out with the voluminous ATPD group. Tables 11.8 and 11.9 report the items and parameters in which the ATPD subgroups differed significantly from the control group with PS. To avoid redundancy, only the significant differences are presented. The numeric values are not repeated but can be found in Chapters 4 to 10. The differences found between the 'voluminous ATPD group' and the control groups were also found within the 'homogeneous ATPD group' – but more accentuated. No additional relevant differences could be recognised.

Analogous to the preceding presentations, Table 11.10 and Table 11.11 report the items and parameters in which the ATPD subgroups differed significantly from the control group with BSAD. Again, to avoid redundancy, only the significant differences are presented. It is a very interesting finding that the 'Acute Schizophrenia-like Psychotic Disorder' does not show any difference to Bipolar Schizoaffective Disorder, especially with regards to prognosis. Perhaps this finding cannot only be singularly explained by acuity and shortness of the psychotic symptomatology. Another important factor determining the similarities between Acute Schizophrenia-like Disorder and Schizoaffective Disorders can be found in their longitudinal syndromatical instability. As previously discussed, many patients who had an Acute Schizophrenia-like Psychotic Disorder as their index episode also showed affective and schizoaffective episodes during course. Thus, they fulfilled the criteria of the so-called sequential type of schizoaffective disorders (see Marneros and Tsuang,

Table 11.8. Significant differences between the voluminous group of ATPD in general, ATPD subgroups and PS (part 1)

	ATPD in general vs. PS	Acute Polymorphic Psychotic Disorder vs. PS	Acute Schizophrenia-like Psychotic Disorder vs. PS
Broken home	–	–	less[c]
High level of education	more[a]	–	more
Premorbid personality obsessoid	more	–	–
Social interactions before onset	more	more[b]	more
Stable heterosexual relationship before onset	more	more	–
Socio-economic status at onset	higher	–	–
Duration of psychotic period	shorter	shorter	shorter
Mode of onset of the acute episode	more acute	more acute	more acute
Life event before onset	more	–	–
Suicidal behaviour during acute episode	less	more	more

[a] Direction of difference when ATPD in general are compared to PS.
[b] Direction of difference when Acute Polymorphic Psychoses are compared to PS.
[c] Direction of difference when Acute Schizophrenia-like Psychoses are compared to PS.

1986; Marneros *et al.*, 1988b,c, 1991b). That is another finding that supports the idea that these disorders are positioned between one end of the psychotic continuum occupied by schizophrenia and the opposite end occupied by major affective disorders. Not only schizoaffective, but also Schizophrenia-like and Polymorphic Psychotic Disorders, could have the function of a bridge between these two ends (see p. 208).

Conclusions: The Acute Polymorphic Psychotic Disorders differ from schizophrenia and schizoaffective disorders in almost the same way as the voluminous Acute and Transient Psychotic Disorder group, but more extensively with regard to outcome (the outcome being more favourable). Acute Schizophrenia-like Psychotic Disorders not only have similarities to schizophrenia but also to schizoaffective disorders, which can probably be explained by their phenomenological instability during long-term course.

Table 11.9. Significant differences between the voluminous group of ATPD in general, ATPD subgroups and PS (part 2)

	ATPD in general vs. PS	Acute Polymorphic Psychotic Disorder vs. PS	Acute Schizophrenia-like Psychotic Disorder vs. PS
GAS at first follow-up	better[a]	better[b]	–
DAS global score at first follow-up	better	better	–
PIRS general score at first follow-up	better	better	–
Disability pension at first follow-up	less	less	less[c]
Stable heterosexual relationship at first follow-up	more	more	–
GAS at end of prospective follow-up	better	better	–
DAS global score at end of prospective follow-up	better	better	–
PANSS positive at end of prospective follow-up	better	better	–
PANSS negative at end of prospective follow-up	better	better	–
Persisting alterations at end of prospective follow-up	less	less	–
Stable heterosexual relationship at end of prospective follow-up	more	more	–
Disability pension at end of prospective follow-up	less	–	–
Full autarky at end of prospective follow-up	more	more	–
Monosyndromal course	less	less	less

[a] Direction of difference when ATPD in general are compared to PS.

[b] Direction of difference when Acute Polymorphic Psychoses are compared to PS.

[c] Direction of difference when Acute Schizophrenia-like Psychoses are compared to PS.

Table 11.10. Significant differences between the voluminous group of ATPD in general, ATPD subgroups and BSAD (part 1)

	ATPD in general vs. BSAD	Acute Polymorphic Psychoses vs. BSAD	Acute Schizophrenia-like Psychosis vs. BSAD
Premorbid personality asthenic/low self-confidence	–	–	more
Stable heterosexual relationship before onset	–	more	–
Age at onset	older[a]	older[b]	–
Duration of psychotic period	shorter	shorter	shorter[c]
Mode of onset of the acute episode	more acute	more acute	more acute
Life event before onset	–	–	more
Suicidal behaviour during whole course of illness	more	–	–

[a] Direction of difference when ATPD in general are compared to BSAD.
[b] Direction of difference when Acute Polymorphic Psychoses are compared to BSAD.
[c] Direction of difference when Acute Schizophrenia-like Psychoses are compared to BSAD.

The relation of cycloid psychoses to ATPD

Although the concept of cycloid psychoses is one of the historical roots of the ICD-10 category of ATPD, identity of the two concepts cannot be taken for granted (Pfuhlmann, 1998; Sigmund and Mundt, 1999). As outlined in Chapter 2, the concept of cycloid psychoses was introduced in 1924 by Karl Kleist (1924), drawing in part on nosological entities described by his teacher Wernicke, such as motility psychosis and anxiety psychosis (Pillmann et al., 2000a; Pillmann and Marneros, 2003). Karl Leonhard later modified the concept and included it in his complex nosological system (Leonhard, 1957, 1999). In this system, the cycloid psychoses comprise three distinct forms of psychoses which have in common a phasic course, remission without residual symptoms and bipolarity: anxiety–elation psychosis, hyperkinetic–akinetic motility psychosis and excited–retarded confusion psychosis. Carlo Perris (1974) confirmed the validity of the concept, but was unable to differentiate Leonard's three subtypes. However, he observed substantial symptomatic overlap. His diagnostic criteria were published in an operational form (Perris and Brockington, 1981; Perris, 1986) (Table 11.12). Perris's investigations further stimulated international interest in the disorder (Cutting et al., 1978; Brockington et al., 1982a). The introduction of ATPD can be seen as an attempt to create a category within ICD-10 to accommodate those patients that would have been diagnosed as having cycloid psychoses in the tradition of Leonhard (1961) and Perris (1974).

Table 11.11. Significant differences between the voluminous group of ATPD in general, ATPD subgroups and BSAD (part 2)

	ATPD in general vs. BSAD	Acute Polymorphic Psychoses vs. BSAD	Acute Schizophrenia-like Psychosis vs. BSAD
GAS at first follow-up	–	better[b]	–
DAS global score at first follow-up	–	–	–
PIRS general score	–	better	–
Disability pension at first follow-up	less[a]	less	–
Stable heterosexual relationship at first follow-up	–	–	–
GAS at end of prospective follow-up	–	better	–
DAS global score at end of prospective follow-up	better	better	–
PANSS positive at end of prospective follow-up	–	–	–
PANSS negative at end of prospective follow-up	–	–	–
Persisting alterations at end of prospective follow-up	–	–	–
Stable heterosexual relationship at end of prospective follow-up	–	–	–
Disability pension at end of prospective follow-up	less	less	–
Full autarky at end of prospective follow-up	–	–	–
Pharmacotherapy at end of prospective follow-up	less	less	–
Annual frequency of episodes	–	–	–
Monosyndromal course	–	–	–

[a] Direction of difference when ATPD in general are compared to BSAD.

[b] Direction of difference when Acute Polymorphic Psychoses are compared to BSAD.

Table 11.12. Cycloid psychosis: definition of Perris and Brockington (1981)

1. An acute psychotic condition, not related to the administration or the abuse of any drug or to brain injury, occurring for the first time in subjects in the age range 15–50 years.
2. The condition has a sudden onset with a rapid change from a state of health to a full-blown psychotic condition within a few hours or at most a very few days.
3. At least four of the following must be present:
    A Confusion of some degree, mostly expressed as perplexity or puzzlement
    B Mood-incongruent delusions of any kind: most often with a persecutory content
    C Hallucinatory experiences of any kind, often related to themes of death
    D An overwhelming, frightening experience of anxiety, not bound to particular situations or circumstances (pan-anxiety)
    E Deep feelings of happiness or ecstasy, most often with a religious colouring
    F Motility disturbances of akinetic or hyperkinetic type which are mostly expressional
    G A particular concern with death
    H Mood swings in the background and not so pronounced to justify a diagnosis of affective disorder.
4. There is no fixed symptomatological combination: on the contrary, the symptomatology may change frequently during the episode and shows a bipolar characteristic.

The ICD-10 criteria of ATPD and the Perris and Brockington definition of cycloid psychosis represent two sets of operational criteria intended to capture the same nosological concept. However, it is not known whether both sets of criteria identify the same patients. The data from the HASBAP have therefore been used to answer two questions: (1) To what extent are the features of ATPD as defined in ICD-10 compatible with the concept of cycloid psychoses? (2) Can cycloid psychoses be regarded as a special subgroup of acute and transient psychoses with particular psychopathological and prognostic features?

The whole group of 42 patients with ATPD was subdivided into those that fulfilled the criteria of Perris and Brockington (Perris and Brockington, 1981; Perris, 1986) for cycloid psychosis during index hospitalisation (the cycloid group) and those who did not (the non-cycloid group).

The main differences and similarities between patients who fulfilled the Perris and Brockington definition of cycloid psychoses and those who did not are shown in Table 11.13. It can be seen that gender distribution did not differentiate between cycloid and non-cycloid ATPD, but abrupt onset and polymorphic features were significantly more common in cycloid than in non-cycloid ATPD. The unification of the ICD-10 categories F23.0 and F23.1 as 'Acute Polymorphic Psychosis' (with or without symptoms of schizophrenia) showed a significant concordance with the diagnosis of cycloid psychosis ($P < 0.02$). With global agreement of 69% and a moderate Cohen's kappa of 0.36, however, concordance was far from perfect.

Table 11.13. Characteristics of 42 patients with Acute and Transient Psychotic Disorders, divided according to a concurrent diagnosis of cycloid psychosis

	Cycloid $n = 23$	Non-cycloid $n = 19$	Statistical analysis
	n (%)	n (%)	P
Gender			
Female	18 (78)	15 (79)	n.s.[a]
Characteristics of the acute episode			
Polymorphic features (F23./1)	19 (83)	9 (47)	0.02[a]
Schizophrenic features (F23.1/2)	12 (52)	13 (68)	n.s.[a]
Abrupt onset (<48 h)	14 (61)	4 (21)	0.01[a]
Acute stress	4 (17)	0 (0)	n.s.[b]
Duration of psychotic symptoms			
Mean ± SD	14.7 ± 11.2 days	20.8 ± 15.1 days	n.s.[c]
Range	1–45 days	1–61 days	
Days in hospital (mean)			
Mean ± SD	39.5 ± 22.1 days	38.8 ± 25.8 days	n.s.[c]
Range	6–86 days	5–94 days	
Course of illness			
Age at first episode			
Mean ± SD	32.1 ± 6.9 years	40.1 ± 13.6 years	0.03[c]
Range	21–45 years	18–70 years	
Age at index episode			
Mean ± SD	39.2 ± 9.8 years	43.7 ± 15.1 years	n.s.[c]
Range	23–61 years	18–73 years	
Number of episodes			
Mean ± SD	3.2 ± 3.7	1.8 ± 1.6	n.s.[c]
Range	1–17	1–7	

[a] χ^2 test.
[b] Fisher's exact test, two-tailed.
[c] t-test.
n.s., no significance.

The data on the index hospitalisation showed only minor differences between the two groups, such as a non-significantly higher frequency of schizophrenic symptoms in the non-cycloid group and a lesser duration of psychotic symptoms and shorter hospital stay for the cycloid group. It has sometimes been assumed that acute and transient psychoses are frequently preceded by acute stress. In the sample of the HASBAP, only four patients fulfilled the ICD-10 criteria of preceding stress, all of them cycloid. Average age at index episode was somewhat lower for cycloid psychosis than for non-cycloid ATPD and age at first episode was 8 years

Table 11.14. Frequency of residual syndromes at follow-up in 38 patients with ATPD, divided according to a concurrent diagnosis of cycloid psychosis. Persisting alterations classified as in Marneros and co-workers (1991b, 1998)

	Cycloid $n = 20$	Non-cycloid $n = 18$	Statistical analysis
	n (%)	n (%)	P
No persisting alterations	15 (75)	9 (50)	n.s.[a]
Slight asthenic insufficiency syndrome	3 (15)	5 (28)	n.s.[b]
Adynamic deficiency syndrome	2 (10)	4 (22)	n.s.[b]

[a] χ^2 test.
[b] Fisher's exact test, two-tailed.
n.s., no significance.

Table 11.15. Outcome measures at follow-up for 38 patients with ATPD, divided according to a concurrent diagnosis of cycloid psychosis

	Cycloid $n = 20$	Non-cycloid $n = 18$	Statistical analysis
	Mean ± SD	Mean ± SD	P^a
Disability Assessment Schedule			
Global score[b]	0.40 ± 0.60	1.28 ± 1.36	0.02
General behaviour subscore[b]	0.54 ± 0.64	1.09 ± 1.33	n.s.
Special roles subscore[b]	0.45 ± 0.67	1.05 ± 0.96	0.03
Psychological Impairments Rating Schedule			
General score[b]	0.15 ± 0.32	0.54 ± 0.61	0.02
Subscore activity/retreat[b]	0.14 ± 0.03	0.50 ± 0.66	0.04
Subscore communication behaviour[b]	0.17 ± 0.35	0.58 ± 0.58	0.02
Global Assessment Scale[c]	86.2 ± 8.2	76.1 ± 19.6	0.054
Range	61–95	35–95	

[a] t-test.
[b] Possible scores range from 0–5, higher scores indicating higher degree of disability/impairment.
[c] Possible scores range from 0–100, higher scores indicating better functioning.
n.s., no significance.

lower for cycloid patients; the latter difference was statistically significant. The non-significantly higher number of episodes (from onset to index episode) in the cycloid group can largely be attributed to the longer observation period.

At the first prospective follow-up interviews conducted between 7 months and 4 years after the index episode, half of the non-cycloid and four-fifths of the cycloid patients were completely free of persisting alterations. The remaining patients showed mild persisting alterations; more severe forms, such as apathetic-paranoid syndrome or chronic psychosis, did not occur (Table 11.14). The differences between cycloid and non-cycloid probands failed to reach statistical significance. WHO/DAS scores as a measure of social disability are given in Table 11.15. With this instrument, the cycloid group showed better social functioning at follow-up both in the global score and in the subscore for special roles. The difference was statistically significant. Similar differences between cycloid and non-cycloid ATPD were demonstrated in psychological impairment (WHO/PIRS) and general level of functioning (GAS) (Table 11.15). The Perris and Brockington definition of cycloid psychosis requires a sudden onset ('within a very few days'), while ICD-10 ATPD may evolve over 14 days. To evaluate the role of the requirement of sudden onset the analyses given in Table 11.15 were therefore repeated with a modified definition of cycloid psychoses that disregarded the onset item. The number of patients considered cycloid according to the modified criterion rose to 29 (69.0%), indicating greater concordance between the diagnosis of ATPD and cycloid psychosis. However, the differences in outcome measures between cycloid and non-cycloid ATPD diminished greatly and were no longer statistically significant (data not shown).

In conclusion, the frequency of ATPD in the HASBAP is lower than the 10–15% of psychotic patients judged to be cycloid by Perris (Perris, 1986), as confirmed by the published figures. For example, Cutting and co-workers (1978) reported an 8%, Leonhard (1995) a 22% and Lindvall (1993) a 24% rate of cycloid psychoses among hospital patients with psychotic disorders. The main reason for the apparently lower frequency of ATPD than of cycloid psychoses is the strict exclusion of patients with major affective episodes and of all patients displaying schizophrenic symptoms for more than a month in the lCD-10 definition of ATPD.

In comparing cycloid and non-cycloid ATPD, both similarities and differences were revealed. There were no differences in gender distribution and the duration of the acute episode did not differ markedly. Cycloid psychoses, however, showed a significantly lower age at first episode. This may be largely a consequence of the age limit included in the Perris and Brockington definition. Although due to the difference in age at onset, total observation time was longer for cycloid psychoses, these patients showed fewer persistent alterations at follow-up, as well as better social adaptation, less psychological impairment and better global functioning. This was documented by significant differences in five of six scales in WHO/DAS and WHO/PIRS and by a difference in GAS that narrowly failed to reach statistical significance. Thus the finding of a good prognosis of cycloid psychoses reported by other authors (Maj, 1988; Beckmann et al., 1990) was confirmed. In addition, it could be shown to hold true in comparison with non-cycloid ATPD. In some cases, cycloid ATPD were associated with acute stress, which was not the case for non-cycloid ATPD.

These findings are also remarkable insofar as an earlier age at onset has been associated with an unfavourable prognosis in predictor studies of psychotic disorders (Davidson and McGlashan, 1997). In contrast, cycloid psychosis has traditionally been regarded as a disorder of young women with a favourable prognosis if frequently recurrent (Kleist, 1928; Perris, 1988). The findings indicate that the operational definition of ATPD by Perris and Brockington (Perris, 1974; Perris and Brockington, 1981) may embrace a subgroup of ATPD that is characterised by earlier onset, frequent recurrence and more favourable prognosis.

It may be asked which of the features that differentiate cycloid psychoses from ATPD in general are responsible for the more favourable prognosis of cycloid psychoses. The features that differentiate the Perris and Brockington definition of cycloid psychoses from the ICD-l0 definition of ATPD are a strict criterion of sudden onset ('within a few days at most') and the presence of a specified symptom set associated with 'cycloid' psychopathology as discussed above. In part, these features are known to be general predictors of good outcome in psychotic disorders; within broad-definition schizophrenic psychosis, for example, good prognostic features including 'sudden onset' and 'confusion' have been described (Robins and Guze, 1970). To elucidate the matter further, a second analysis of the data was conducted, which showed the requirement of sudden onset included in the definition of cycloid psychosis to be very largely responsible for its predictive value. With this qualification in mind, it should be noted that previous predictor studies have focussed on schizophrenia. To date, no predictors have been demonstrated in ATPD. The HASBAP showed that even in this group, highly selected for rapid onset and short duration as it is, a diagnosis of cycloid psychosis as defined by Perris and Brockington seems to be of prognostic value.

> Conclusion: There is a considerable concordance of cycloid psychoses and the polymorphic subtype of Acute and Transient Psychotic Disorders.

The relation of bouffée délirante to ATPD

As described in detail on page 24ff, the most ancient – and certainly a very influential – source for ICD-10 ATPD is the concept of 'bouffée délirante'. Today, bouffée délirante has its place in French psychiatry as documented by its inclusion in the national classification system INSERM (1969) and the formulation of operational criteria by Pull and co-workers (Pull et al., 1983, 1984; Pichot, 1986a). Mainly in France and Francophone countries, case reports, theoretical articles and clinical studies continue to be published.

Although the bouffée délirante played an important role in the creation of ICD-10 ATPD, little is known regarding the concordance of ICD-10 ATPD and bouffée délirante. In order to investigate the relationship of ATPD and bouffée délirante, an analysis of the HASBAP data compared patients with ATPD that concurrently fulfilled the criteria of bouffée délirante with those who did not (Pillmann *et al.*, 2003). In this analysis, two questions were addressed: (1) What concordance exists between the ICD-10 diagnosis of ATPD and a diagnosis of bouffée délirante? (2) Do patients with bouffée délirante differ in prognosis from other patients with ATPD?

When diagnosed according to the criteria of Pull and co-workers (1983), only a minority of cases ($n = 12$) was classified as bouffée délirante. This was 28.6% of all patients with ATPD, 1.2% of all patients treated for non-organic psychotic or major affective disorders (F2 or F3 of ICD-10) during the study period or 2.4% of all patients treated for nonorganic psychotic disorders (F2 of ICD-10). Ten (83.3%) of 12 patients with bouffée délirante belonged to the polymorphic subtype of ATPD, while among the 30 patients with ATPD not fulfilling the criteria of bouffée délirante, 18 (60%) belonged to the polymorphic subtype. Thus nearly all patients with bouffée délirante belonged to the polymorphic subtype of ATPD. However, many patients with a polymorphic subtype of ATPD did not meet the Pull and co-workers criteria of bouffée délirante. Thus, concordance between the two diagnoses is far from complete. Bouffée délirante as operationally diagnosed can best be described as a subgroup of ATPD, but much less voluminous.

For further analysis, the sample was divided into two groups: those patients that fulfilled the Pull and co-workers (1983) criteria of bouffée délirante and those that did not. None of the parameters of the acute episode differentiated significantly between bouffée délirante and non-bouffée délirante. Associated acute stress showed a tendency to be more frequent in bouffée délirante patients with Acute Schizophrenia-like Psychoses (Pillmann *et al.*, 2003). The only significant difference between patients with bouffée délirante and those without concerned age. In bouffée délirante, age at onset and age at index episode were lower. This difference is compatible with the operational definition of bouffée délirante, which demands onset until approximately 40 years of age. In contrast, in ATPD onset was not restricted to any specific age group but could occur as late as age 70 years. No differences were found in course parameters between bouffée délirante and non-bouffée délirante patients (Pillmann *et al.*, 2003).

Tables 11.16 and 11.17 give course and outcome parameters until the first follow-up for the bouffée délirante and the non-bouffée délirante samples. (For details see Pillmann *et al.*, 2003). The number of relapses did not differ significantly between the bouffée délirante sample and the non-bouffée délirante sample.

Table 11.16 gives a number of psychosocial variables as markers of psychosocial functioning and treatment status. Although – consistent with the considerable

Table 11.16. Psychosocial parameters at follow-up in 12 patients with bouffée délirante compared to 30 patients with ATPD not fulfilling the criteria of bouffée délirante (non-bouffée délirante)

	Bouffée délirante $n = 12$	Non-bouffée délirante $n = 26$	Statistical analysis
	n (%)	n (%)	P
Employed	9 (75.0)	9 (34.6)	0.020[a]
Stable heterosexual partnership	10 (83.3)	13 (50.0)	0.077[b]
On psychiatric medication	7 (58.3)	21 (80.8)	0.253[b]
Autark (living independently)	1 (8.3)	2 (7.7)	1.000[b]

[a] χ^2 test.
[b] Fisher's exact test, two-tailed.

Table 11.17. Outcome measures at follow-up in 12 patients with bouffée délirante compared to 30 patients with ATPD not fulfilling the criteria of bouffée délirante (non-bouffée délirante)

	Bouffée délirante $n = 12$	Non-bouffée délirante $n = 26$	Statistical analysis
	Mean ± SD	Mean ± SD	P
Disability Assessment Schedule			
Global score[a]	0.67 ± 0.98	0.88 ± 1.18	0.581[d]
General behaviour subscore[a]	0.67 ± 0.89	0.87 ± 1.12	0.594[d]
Special roles subscore[a]	0.49 ± 0.86	0.84 ± 0.86	0.250[d]
Psychological Impairments Rating Schedule			
General score[a]	0.26 ± 0.46	0.38 ± 0.54	0.510[d]
Subscore activity/retreat[a]	0.23 ± 0.42	0.35 ± 0.58	0.547[d]
Subscore communication behaviour[a]	0.28 ± 0.52	0.40 ± 0.57	0.522[d]
Global Assessment Score (mean values)[b]	83.4 ± 15.4	80.5 ± 15.6	0.594[d]
GAS > 70 (n, %)	11 (91.7)	21 (80.8)	0.643[c]

[a] Scores are on a scale ranging from 0 to 5, higher scores indicating greater disability/impairment.
[b] Scores are on a scale ranging from 1 to 100, higher scores indicating higher level of functioning.
[c] Fisher's exact test, two-tailed.
[d] t-test, two-tailed.

relapse rate – most patients were on psychotropic (mainly antipsychotic) medication at follow-up, they showed high rates of stable partnership and employment, and nearly all patients could live independently in the community. Interestingly, patients with bouffée délirante were significantly more frequently employed at follow-up than patients without a diagnosis of bouffée délirante. The difference diminished only slightly when patients older than 60 years were excluded from the analysis. Patients with bouffée délirante were also more often in a stable heterosexual partnership at follow-up and less often on medication, but the differences were not statistically significant. WHO/DAS scores as a measure of social disability are given in Table 11.17. Mean scores were calculated, with a higher score indicating a greater degree of handicap. There were no significant differences between bouffée délirante and non-bouffée délirante patients in WHO/DAS, WHO/PIRS and GAS scores. However, in all measures there was a slight advantage of the bouffée délirante group. In general, the outcome was favourable; 11 of the patients with bouffée délirante (91.7%) and 20 of the patients without bouffée délirante (80.8%) showed a GAS score greater than 70 at follow-up.

The fact that only 28.6% of the patients with ATPD were concurrently diagnosed as bouffée délirante shows that the operational definition of bouffée délirante is much narrower than that of ATPD. Even ATPD in the sample of the HASBAP was relatively rare and amounted to only 4.1% of all inpatients with non-organic psychotic or major affective episodes, or 8.5% of all patients with non-organic psychotic episodes. In consequence, patients with bouffée délirante in this sample only represent 1.2% or 2.4%, respectively. This finding is in contrast to the fact that bouffée délirante remains a popular diagnosis among French clinicians (Pichot, 1982; Ferrey and Zebdi, 1999) applying to approximately 16% of psychotic patients (Johnson-Sabine et al., 1983). However, the diagnosis seems to be less frequent in research settings (Johnson-Sabine et al., 1983). Singer and co-workers (1980), in their follow-up investigation of 74 patients initially diagnosed with bouffée délirante, already noted that only a narrow subgroup of patients ($n = 19$) fulfilled the strict criteria of Pichot (1979). Also taking into account the follow-up data, these authors concluded that only 0.47% of psychiatric admissions were 'true' bouffées délirantes. The criteria suggested by Pull and co-workers (1983) require, among others, acute onset, a specified polymorphic syndrome, full remission and absence of different psychotic episodes, all of these obligatory. While these criteria were derived from the empirical study of the diagnostic practice of French psychiatrists, it seems that in everyday use, the criteria are followed less strictly than an operational procedure would require.

As the operational criteria for bouffée délirante result in a narrow selection of patients, the question arises whether these patients are also selected for a particularly favourable prognosis. There is indeed some indication that this is the case. Patients with bouffée délirante were significantly more often employed at follow-up, they were more often in a stable heterosexual partnership and they showed a slightly more favourable outcome on most standardised outcome scales. The small number of subjects did not allow, however, these differences to be confirmed statistically.

The problem of low statistical power is not particular to the HASBAP, but results from the low incidence of operationally diagnosed bouffée délirante as discussed above. Since the samples of the HASBAP were selected from 1036 inpatients, a study with a higher statistical power would need to screen a very high number of patients.

The following considerations argue for the validity of these findings. Firstly, there is a strong converging trend in the outcome measures pointing in the direction of a more favourable prognosis of bouffée délirante. Secondly, the findings are compatible with results from a separate analysis of the HASBAP. This analysis showed that a concurrent diagnosis of cycloid psychosis (which also includes a polymorphic symptom picture and sudden onset as defining criteria) also carried the implication of a more favourable prognosis (Pillmann et al., 2001) (see page 191). Thirdly, the findings are concordant with the study of Singer and co-workers (1980). These authors analysed the course in 19 patients diagnosed with bouffée délirante according to Pichot (1979) and contrasted the results with 28 patients diagnosed with bouffée délirante on clinical grounds. They noted that evolution towards schizophrenia was less common in narrowly diagnosed bouffée délirante.

Conclusion: Although bouffées délirantes show substantial overlaps with Acute and Transient Psychotic Disorders, they are more narrowly defined so they have a considerably lower incidence than Acute and Transient Psychotic Disorders when diagnosed with operational criteria. Most of them belong to the polymorphic group of Acute and Transient Psychotic Disorders. The diagnosis, therefore, can be fully integrated into the Polymorphic subgroup of Acute and Transient Psychotic Disorders, so that no necessity exists for a separate diagnosis of 'bouffée délirante'.

12

What are brief, acute and transient psychotic disorders?

In the introduction to the present book, we compared the efforts of psychiatrists to define homogeneous groups of mental disorders with the work of a sculptor working with clay. Like the artist, who usually has to cut small, but also sometimes larger pieces of wood, marble or clay in an attempt to give material an identifiable feature, so the psychiatrist has to exclude smaller groups with 'atypical' features from the larger groups of 'typical disorders'. But, the small atypical groups of mental disorders excluded from the large groups of typical disorders continue to exist; just as the left-over material of the sculpture which has been cut continues to exist – not as part of the sculpture, but rather as material left in the sculptor's workshop.

The creation by the WHO of the category F23 in the ICD-10 (i.e. the category 'Acute and Transient Psychotic Disorder') reflects the efforts of the psychiatrists to gather together parts of the excluded material remaining after forming the big category of schizophrenia – together with another uncertain mass, namely 'schizoaffective disorder'. The DSM-IV group of 'Brief Psychosis' is, as we show, part of the ICD-10 Acute and Transient Psychotic Disorders category. Psychotic disorder with acute onset, short duration and usually dramatic polymorphic symptomatology – already described and classified within the framework of more or less national concepts in many countries – belong in this new category of ICD-10, as we pointed out in Chapters 1 and 2. But the WHO, in spite of creating this new category, remains uncertain regarding its correctness: '*The nomenclature of these acute disorders is as uncertain as their nosological status [. . .] Systematic clinical information that would provide definitive guidance on the classification of acute psychotic disorders is not yet available, and the limited data and clinical tradition that must therefore be used instead do not give rise to concepts that can be clearly defined and separated from each other*' *(WHO 1992)*. This is quite true, but also a challenge for research on the topic. That was also the reason to design and carry out the Halle Study on Brief and Acute Psychoses (HASBAP).

Do the findings of the HASBAP and those of other studies on Brief and Acute Psychoses give answers to important questions connected with the topic? Do the facts and data diminish some of the uncertainties mentioned by the WHO? We believe the answer to both questions is yes, at least partially. But perhaps more important is the possibility that these studies may give some stimulation for future clinical, biological or genetic research.

The answers to the main questions and the resulting considerations are:

What are Acute and Transient Psychotic Disorders?

Acute and Transient Psychotic Disorder, as defined by the ICD-10 involving also the 'Brief Psychoses' of DSM-IV, are disorders:
- mainly concerning females,
- with possible onset in all ages of adult life, but usually between the thirtieth and fiftieth year of life,
- having an acute or even abrupt onset,
- whose onset is only rarely dependent on acute severe stress,
- with a very short psychotic period,
- in which stressful events are only rarely associated immediately with the onset of episodes,
- with a very good response to antipsychotic drugs, and
- with a usually favourable outcome, in spite of the fact that they are usually recurrent.

How can people suffering from Acute and Transient Psychotic Disorders be described?

A majority of patients with Acute and Transient Psychotic Disorders have an education, occupational status and level of functioning with no significant differences from the mentally healthy population. They also have an average level of social interaction and activities, as well as the same frequency of stable heterosexual partnerships as mentally healthy people do. But, because of the recurrence of their illness, it is possible in some socio-economic systems, especially in times of high unemployment, to be excluded from the labour market. But, nevertheless, even in such situations, they do not usually lose their autarky.

Are there any significant differences from typical schizophrenia and schizoaffective disorders?

Gender

An important characteristic of ATPD concerns gender. The vast majority of patients with Acute and Transient Psychotic Disorders are females, while the gender distribution in schizophrenia and Bipolar Schizoaffective Disorders is almost equal (Dohrenwend and Dohrenwend, 1976; Munk-Jørgensen, 1985; Schubart, 1986; Häfner, 1987; Lewine, 1988; Marneros *et al.*, 1990b, 1991b; Leung and Chue, 2000). In the HASBAP, the comparative groups to Acute and Transient Psychotic Disorders, namely schizophrenia and schizoaffective disorders, are matched regarding gender and age. However, based on the findings of the international literature cited above, it can be said that Acute and Transient Psychotic Disorders differ from schizophrenia and Bipolar Schizoaffective Disorders regarding gender distribution.

Age at onset

It also seems that the age at onset in Acute and Transient Psychotic Disorders patients is higher than in schizophrenic and bipolar schizoaffective patients. The HASBAP found a difference in age at onset between Acute and Transient Psychotic Disorders and Bipolar Schizoaffective Disorder, but not between Acute and Transient Psychotic Disorders and Positive Schizophrenia. We think that this is an artificial finding, which depends on the selection of the group of schizophrenic patients. The patients were patients with so-called 'positive' schizophrenia (which is assumed to have a higher age at onset than schizophrenia with mainly 'negative' symptomatology, see Marneros *et al.*, 1991b; Häfner *et al.*, 1991). The second cause is that the vast majority of the schizophrenic group has to be female due to the matched design of the study. But it is also well known that the age at onset of schizophrenia in females is higher than in males (Lewine, 1988; Häfner *et al.*, 1989; Häfner and an der Heiden, 1997; Leung and Chue, 2000). Thus, when the epidemiological literature is taken into account, the age at onset of Acute and Transient Psychotic Disorders appears to be higher than that of schizophrenia and much higher than that of Bipolar Schizoaffective Disorder.

Premorbid features

With regard to premorbid adaptation, social interactions, achievement and social status, Acute and Transient Psychotic Disorders patients do not differ significantly from mentally healthy people. In contrast, they show marked differences to patients with schizophrenia in these domains. The differences from patients with schizoaffective disorder are only partial and, all in all, subtle.

Symptomatology

In the domain of symptomatology, the Acute and Transient Psychotic Disorders differ from both schizophrenia and Bipolar Schizoaffective Disorders mainly through the rapidly changing delusional topics, the more frequent occurrence of anxiety and the rapid change of mood states. As could be expected, with regard to the bipolarity of symptomatology, within the episode, Acute and Transient Psychotic Disorders differ from schizophrenia but not from schizoaffective disorders, especially from their mixed type.

Features of episodes

The abrupt onset, the shorter psychotic period and shorter duration of the episode are additional differentiating features between Acute and Transient Psychotic Disorder and schizophrenia on the one hand, and schizoaffective disorders, on the other hand.

Precipitating factors

The ICD-10 specifier 'associated acute stress' is useless as defined in ICD-10. It seems to be a rare phenomenon in Acute and Transient Psychotic Disorder. Its specifying power for Acute and Transient Psychotic Disorders should be re-considered. However, the importance of precipitating factors in Acute and Transient Psychotic Disorders depends on the criteria used. It may be more useful to extend the time period for the coding of acute stress to life events during a longer period and to include mildly or moderately stressful events. Such events more often precede Acute and Transient Psychotic Disorders than schizophrenic episodes. But, even then, a stressful life event is not characteristic for the majority of Acute and Transient Psychotic Disorders. Most importantly: the presence of a preceding life event seems to carry no prognostic significance in Acute and Transient Psychotic Disorder.

Syndrome stability during course

One of the most important differences between Acute and Transient Psychotic Disorders, Positive Schizophrenia and Bipolar Schizoaffective Disorder is the great stability of schizophrenic syndromes on the one hand, and the great instability of the schizoaffective syndromes, on the other. Acute and Transient Psychotic Disorders occupy a position between the two other psychotic groups. But one of the most interesting findings is that – if the group of Schizophrenia-like Psychoses is excluded – none of the patients with Acute and Transient Psychotic Disorders changed during the prospective follow-up period into schizophrenia, but some of them changed into schizoaffective or affective disorder.

Outcome

Regarding the outcome variables, it can be said that patients with Acute and Transient Psychotic Disorders have the best global functioning at the end of the observation time with significant differences to schizophrenia, but only slight differences to schizoaffective disorders. The same can be said regarding social consequences of the illness like disability pension, autarky, occupational status and stable heterosexual partnerships. But it seems that all three kinds of psychotic disorders need long-term pharmacotherapy, especially antipsychotics. Patients with Bipolar Schizoaffective Disorders, and some patients with Acute and Transient Psychotic Disorders, also require mood stabilisers.

Summarising the above findings it can be said that yes, there are some significant differences between the Acute and Transient Psychotic Disorders and schizophrenia regarding:
- gender distribution,
- age at onset,
- premorbid level of functioning and premorbid social interactions,
- onset, development, duration and phenomenology, as well as structure of symptomatology,
- level of postepisodic functioning and outcome in general.
- But it seems that a subgroup of Acute and Transient Psychotic Disorders – the 'Acute Schizophrenia-like Psychoses' – have a closer relationship to Schizophrenia and Schizoaffective Disorders.

It can also be said that:

The differences between Acute and Transient Psychotic Disorders and schizoaffective disorders, especially their bipolar type, are fewer than between Acute and Transient Psychotic Disorders and schizophrenia. Indeed, there are many more similarities. They differ with regard to:
- gender,
- age at onset,
- mode of onset,
- duration and phenomenology, as well as structure of symptomatology.
But Acute and Transient Psychotic Disorders and schizoaffective disorders have strong similarities regarding:
- premorbid level of functioning,
- premorbid interactions and outcome.
- It is also remarkable that in the longitudinal course of patients with Acute and Transient Psychotic Disorders, affective and schizoaffective episodes occur relatively frequently, showing similarities to the course of schizoaffective disorder.

Is the category of 'Acute and Transient Psychotic Disorders' with its subcategories in its present form as defined by the WHO justified?

- The Acute Schizophrenia-like Psychoses probably do not belong to this category, but rather to schizophrenia, or the sequential type of schizoaffective disorder. Perhaps they should best be allocated to a category 'for further research'.
- The distinction of Acute Polymorphic Psychotic Disorders into the group 'with symptoms of schizophrenia' (F23.0) and into the group 'without symptoms of schizophrenia' (F23.1) is unwarranted. There are no differences between the two groups. And, therefore, there is no reason at all to separate them.
- The recent findings support the opinion that in its present form the category of Acute and Transient Psychotic Disorders is not justified.
- But if 'Schizophrenia-like Psychoses' are excluded from category F23, the remaining disorders are almost only the polymorphic type, which is the core type of Acute and Transient Psychotic Disorders. The polymorphism of symptomatology characterised by rapidly changing mood and very unstable psychotic topics obviously has a differentiating and prognostic relevance – it seems to be the essential feature of category F23. So, the correct nomenclature or the category should be '**Brief Polymorphic Psychoses**'.

Are the 'Acute and Transient Psychotic Disorders' or the 'Brief Polymorphic Psychoses' an independent nosological entity?

The above question has to be put dichotomically in the following sense:

1. Are the Acute and Transient Psychotic Disorders – especially their core subgroup, the 'Brief Polymorphic Psychoses' – an independent nosological entity?
2. If not, do they have relevant special features justifying a special clinical and research position?

The question of the nosological independence of the Acute and Transient Psychotic Disorders in general, and also of their core group – the Brief Polymorphic Psychoses – must be rejected!

Not only due to the many and relevant overlaps with schizophrenia and schizoaffective disorders, but also due to affective groups, especially their 'mixed states', and mainly because of their syndromatic instability. Even if the group of

'Schizophrenia-like Psychoses' is excluded (and if only the more homogeneous group of 'Acute Polymorphic Psychoses' is considered), then it is shown that **60% of patients with more than one episode have other kinds of episodes than Acute and Transient Psychotic episodes during course especially affective and schizoaffective.** The changeability of the type of episodes during course, namely the manifestation of episodes belonging to other major disorders is one of the most important arguments – although not the only one – against the assumption that Acute and Transient Psychotic Disorders, or their subgroup 'Acute Polymorphic Psychoses', are a separate nosological entity.

The same findings (i.e. family, premorbidity, course, kind of episode, and outcome data) support the assumption that the 'Brief Polymorphic Psychoses' are also related to the affective spectrum.

Considering the similarities between the 'Brief Polymorphic Psychoses' – the core group of 'Acute and Transient Psychotic Disorders' – and the 'Cycloid Psychotic Disorders', the findings reported in the literature can be mutually transferred from the one to the other diagnostic group.

The findings reported do not bear out the assumption of some authors (Beckmann and Franzek, 2001) that the so-called 'cycloid psychoses' are an independent nosological entity. On the basis of the Leonhard classification (Leonhard, 1957) and supported by their twin investigations, as well as their prognostic findings, the above-mentioned authors and their group concluded that the schizophrenic spectrum can be divided into three large subgroups: 'cycloid psychoses', 'unsystematic' and 'systematic' schizophrenia (Beckmann *et al.*, 1990, 2000; Beckmann and Franzek, 2001; Franzek and Beckmann, 1998a). Of these subgroups, the 'cycloid psychoses' are, as already mentioned, essentially concordant with the 'Acute Polymorphic Psychotic Disorders' of the ICD-10 (Pillmann *et al.*, 2001) – or, at least according to the opinion of the above group, they show considerable overlap (Beckmann and Franzek, 2001).

However, the position that within the groups of psychoses having schizophrenic symptoms, no continuum exists, but rather exactly separated entities, could not be confirmed by the studies concerning Acute and Transient Psychotic Disorders. On the contrary, they support findings from various domains of psychiatry, demonstrating significant overlaps between schizophrenia, affective and schizoaffective disorders (Angst, 1995; Crow, 1995; Mundt, 1995; Marneros *et al.*, 1995b; Crow, 2000; for overview see Marneros *et al.*, 1995a).

> Thus, psychopathology alone, especially the psychopathology of single episodes, cannot be the basis for nosological categorisation. If psychopathology is forced to comply with the postulated categorisations, overexact dogmatic differentiations occur. And then, as Mundt (1995) pointed out, they force clinical reality into a straitjacket. *It can also be said that on the single-symptom level in general, no specificity for psychotic disorders and, thus, no single-disease entity can be found within the spectrum of the functional (or idiopathic or endogenous) psychoses).*

Rejecting the case of the independence of 'Acute and Transient Psychotic Disorders', we have to answer the following question:

Do the Acute and Transient Psychotic Disorders have relevant special features justifying a special clinical and research position?

> Yes, there are a lot of special features characterising the entire group of Acute and Transient Psychotic Disorders as well as the core group 'Acute Polymorphic Psychoses' as is reported in this book. But not all of them are the characteristics of every individual patient suffering from the core group Acute and Transient Psychotic Disorders, or even of every individual patient suffering from 'Acute Polymorphic Psychosis'. A variety of individual features exists. But, nevertheless, the majority of the patients occupy a special position, not identical to schizophrenia, schizoaffective or affective disorders.

From a statistical point of view, patients with Acute and Transient Psychotic Disorders are people with good premorbid adaptation, an acute and usually dramatic, but short-term psychotic symptomatology, and good prognosis. They need acute and immediate psychopharmacological treatment, especially with antipsychotics and possibly – in view of the high recurrence of illness and its relationship to affective disorders – prophylaxis with a mood stabiliser. In this sense, they are in fact a special group. The diagnosis 'Acute and Transient Psychotic Disorders' or 'Brief Polymorphic Psychosis' can mean for patients a hope of a favourable outcome and a low probability of developing deficits, personality changes, difficulties in social interactions, or loss of autarky.

The findings discussed in this book do not support an absolutely favourable outcome with a 'lack of affective or behavioural defective states in *literally all patients*' as Beckmann and co-workers (1990) reported for 'cycloid' patients. Even the polymorphic group of Acute and Transient Psychotic Disorders, with its high concordance with the cycloid disorders, have in 20% of the patients deficits and persisting alterations. The findings of the HASBAP confirm the findings of other studies showing that not all patients with 'cycloid psychoses' have a constitutio at integrum (Perris, 1974; Brockington *et al.*, 1982a; Maj, 1990a). But the same findings, as well as those of the HASBAP, support the thesis that the cycloid symptomatology has a very strong prognostic validity in the sense of a favourable outcome. Perhaps it could be assumed that the 'polymorphic' or 'cycloid' symptomatology could have a partially different neurophysiological background than core schizophrenia, which also has a significant impact on outcome as Sigmund and Mundt (1999) hypothesised.

One of the most powerful arguments against the nosological entity of Brief Polymorphic Psychoses is their longitudinal instability and changeability: they can change over the long term into other phenomenological types like major depression, mania, schizodepression, schizomania or mixed states. The syndromal stability longitudinally is present only in cases at the ends of the spectrum as Angst (1995) remarked. In the centre, where schizoaffective states are located, continued Angst, there is high instability at the psychopathological level. This is also true for the Brief Polymorphic Psychosis.

But, nevertheless, the separation of the Acute and Transient Psychotic Disorders, especially the 'Brief Polymorphic Psychoses', from the core group of schizophrenia is, in spite of their unclear nosological position, not only necessary because of its relevance in the creation of homogeneous groups for research purposes, but also for comparative studies, especially in genetics and biology. It may also be a stimulation for a better understanding of the neurophysiological background of the psychotic disorders and the bridge between them.

13

Brief polymorphic psychoses as a component of a psychotic continuum

Diagnosis is a central task in psychiatry – clinically, determining the approach to treatment and the prognosis, and in research, identifying the population of interest. However, psychiatric diagnoses are based solely on clinical grounds with no external validating parameters. Furthermore, there are several determinants driving current diagnostic practice that may not be helpful to the needs of genetic and biological research (Crow, 1995; Mundt, 1995; Marneros *et al.*, 1995a; Duffy and Grof, 2001).

Disease entities have to be determined by identical symptoms, course, aetiology and pathomorphology. The research process is meant to follow a constant approximation of this idea. Hence, as Mundt (1995) pointed out, outlining perspectives from a mere psychopathological point of view is a difficult task, since psychopathological validation of nosological concepts usually implies external validation with course, outcome, biological parameters, genetics and personality, and will probably result in outlining a type of mental disorganisation, perhaps inherent with its structure, rather than producing stringent mental concomitants of particular biological disturbances. Conventions rather than objective findings mark the borders, whereas only the extremes are very discriminating. It is therefore not surprising that the debate concerning the controversy of psychotic continuum versus separate entity is as old as the scientific psychiatry itself (Berrios and Beer, 1994).

A clear-cut dichotomy between schizophrenia and mood disorders – the two biggest and classical pillars of the so-called idiopathic or endogenous psychoses – does not exist. Even Kraepelin, the creator of the dichotomy of the psychoses, noted it in 1920. Yet, there are no specific findings correlated only with schizophrenia or mood disorders in all possible domains (Carpenter *et al.*, 1995), such as psychopathology (Mundt, 1995), prognosis (Marneros *et al.*, 1995b), genetics (Tsuang, 1995), psychopharmacology (Meltzer, 1995), neuroimaging (Andreasen and Flaum, 1995), biochemistry (van Kammen, 1995), histological (Benes, 1995) or other domains (Angst, 1995; Crow, 1995).

Perhaps this is not the result of our possible insufficient methods of research, but the very nature of mental disorders. Obviously, the recognition of mental disorders not belonging to the core of schizophrenia or mood disorders is not only a function of differing phenomenology, but also of many other factors like prognosis, gender distribution, family and genetics. The schizoaffective disorders have the most prominent position within the group of non-typical non-core schizophrenia. The reason is that schizoaffective disorders challenge the dichotomy concept of schizophrenia vs. mood disorders very radically through the presence of the characteristics of both groups, which theoretically have to be mutually excluded. Together with the fact they are not rare, this is one of the possible explanations for why the nosological position of schizoaffective disorders has been intensively and controversially discussed (Maj, 1984; see also contributions in Marneros and Tsuang, 1986, 1990; Marneros *et al.*, 1995a; Marneros and Goodwin, 2004).

But, as the World Health Organization complains, the Brief Polymorphic Psychoses, or whatever they are called, have only rarely been a focus of research interest. The reasons for this are perhaps that they are less frequent than schizoaffective disorders and that the contrast in the symptomatology is not very obvious. Their psychotic symptomatology and good prognosis led to labels like 'good prognosis' or 'remitting schizophrenia', which is a very superficial solution. But also putting them as ICD-10 and DSM-IV did, into a 'schizophrenic spectrum', is not rational. For schizoaffective psychoses, it is evident that their relationship to mood disorders is perhaps much closer than to schizophrenia. But, nevertheless, they share features and findings of both disorders, schizophrenia and mood disorders. In this sense, it has been assumed that schizoaffective disorders belong to a psychotic continuum extending between schizophrenic and mood disorders (Marneros *et al.*, 1995a,b). But for the Brief Polymorphic Psychosis, no similar discussion or proposal exists. In contrast, the creators and main presenters of a concept of non-schizophrenic Brief Polymorphic Psychosis, like Wernicke, Kleist and Leonhard, as well as their epigones, absolutely confirmed in an almost religious dogmatism that this group of psychosis is an independent nosological entity.

But the early research on the topic, unfortunately yet rare and somewhat unsystematic, and especially the Halle Study on Brief and Acute Psychoses (HASBAP), which is the most voluminous and most systematic comparative study on the topic, cannot confirm the assumption of an independent nosological entity. Rather, the overlaps between Brief Polymorphic Psychosis and schizophrenia on the one hand, and Brief Polymorphic Disorders, schizoaffective and mood disorders (especially their mixed forms) on the other hand, are considerable. It seems that Brief Polymorphic Psychoses cannot be assumed to be a subgroup of schizophrenia. But neither are they a group of a so-called schizophrenic spectrum, whatever this means. There is also no reliable definition of the elastic and changeable schizophrenic spectrum (Andreasen and Flaum, 1995), nor is there a reliable definition of the elastic and

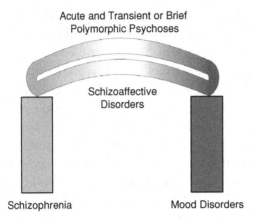

Fig. 13.1.   Brief Polymorphic Psychoses and Schizoaffective Disorders as part of a psychotic continuum.

changeable 'affective spectrum' (Akiskal and Pinto, 2000). If we accept a continuity between the various psychotic groups – but not only between them – then the position of the Brief Polymorphic Psychosis is obviously a position within the spectrum of the psychotic continuum. The research findings up to date reject the idea that schizoaffective disorders and Brief Polymorphic Disorders are identical, which means they do not comprise a single bridge between schizophrenia and affective disorders. Instead, they connect not only the two classical mental disorders, but also the connections and relations with one another. There is namely a continuum within the continuum (see Fig. 13.1).

The following recommendations and remarks of Duffy and Grof (2001) could be also our recommendations and answer to the question: What shall we do with the cases-in-between such as 'Brief Polymorphic Psychoses?' Our psychiatric forefathers, such as Emil Kraepelin and Eugen Bleuler, were clinicians developing psychiatric diagnoses for the purpose of clinical description and clinical communication. When psychiatric research strengthened in the 1960s, operationalised diagnostic criteria for research were developed. But when the research criteria were 'converted' by a group of committees into the DSM and ICD, we were given a system that tried to serve everyone: clinicians, psychiatric statisticians, administrators, insurance companies and others. As pointed out by Angst and Ernst (1993), we need to collect research data and develop diagnostic strategies independent of current diagnostic trends so that the value of this data will remain intact while the diagnostic fashion changes. The task of defining a phenotype closely tied to the underlying genes is further complicated by the existence of phenocopies (non-genetically based forms of the illness) and variable presentations of the disease genotype within and between affected individuals, possibly reflecting epistasis. Therefore, genetic studies require a conservative phenotype definition to be rigorously applied in order to identify a homogeneous subgroup of patients who likely share the same susceptibility genes. It is important to realise the limitations of our current diagnostic approach. We can hardly expect to find genes for a disorder unless the phenotypic description is reasonably valid, reliable and stable. Unfortunately, our profession has developed a habit of using the same diagnostic strategy toward very different ends. Research, treatment, statistics for public health tasks and disability pensions are all very different activities. What fits one will not well suit another. For example, while public health statistics seek to categorise every case, research usually requires exclusivity via selection/exclusion criteria in order to achieve homogeneity (Duffy and Grof, 2001).

Conclusion: The exclusion of a group of 'Brief Polymorphic Psychoses' from the group of schizophrenia, schizoaffective or affective disorders is strongly recommended for research and clinical purposes. Our final recommendation: The Acute and Transient Psychotic Disorders have to be defined according to their decisive characteristic, namely the polymorphic and brief symptomatology. Disorders, which do not meet this essential characteristic, do not belong to this group. They are obviously not an autonomous nosological entity. But also a defined group of 'Brief Polymorphic Psychoses' in spite of its overlap with schizophrenia, schizoaffective or mood disorders has to be considered exclusively for clinical and research purposes, since the Delphic oracle of their nature and that of all psychotic disorders in general, is still unsolved.

References

Abe, S., Suzuki, T., Hori, T., Baba, A. and Shiraishi, H. (1998). Hypogammaglobulinemia during antipsychotic therapy. *Psychiatry and Clinical Neurosciences*, **52**, 115–117.

Ackerknecht, E. H. (1968). A Short History of Psychiatry, 2nd rev. edn. New York: Hafner.

Agid, O., Shapira, B., Zislin, J. *et al.* (1999). Environment and vulnerability to major psychiatric illness: a case control study of early parental loss in major depression, bipolar disorder and schizophrenia. *Molecular Psychiatry*, **4**, 163–172.

Akiskal, H. S. (1989). New insights into the nature and heterogeneity of mood disorders. *Journal of Clinical Psychiatry*, **50** (Suppl.), 6–10; discussion 11–12.

Akiskal, H. S. and Pinto, O. (2000). The soft bipolar spectrum: footnotes to Kraepelin on the interface of hypomania, temperament and depression. In *Bipolar Disorders. 100 Years After Manic-depressive Insanity*, ed. A. Marneros and J. Angst. Dordrecht, Boston, London: Kluwer, pp. 37–62.

Albus, M., Strauss, A. and Stieglitz, R. D. (1990). Schizophrenia, schizotypal and delusional disorders (section F2): results of the ICD-10 field trial. *Pharmacopsychiatry*, **23** (Suppl. 4), 155–159.

Alexander, F. and Selesnick, S. T. (1966). *The History of Psychiatry: An Evaluation of Psychiatric Thought and Practice from Prehistoric Times to the Present*. New York: Harper & Row.

Allodi, F. (1982). Acute paranoid reaction (bouffée délirante) in Canada. *Canadian Journal of Psychiatry*, **27**, 366–373.

Amador, X. F., Friedman, J. H., Kasapis, C., Yale, S. A., Flaum, M. and Gorman, J. M. (1996). Suicidal behavior in schizophrenia and its relationship to awareness of illness. *American Journal of Psychiatry*, **153**, 1185–1188.

AMDP (1995). *Arbeitsgemeinschaft für Methodik und Dokumentation in der Psychiatrie: Das AMDP-System: Manual zur Dokumentation psychiatrischer Befunde. 5. Auflage*. Göttingen: Hogrefe.

Amin, S., Singh, S. P., Brewin, J., Jones, P. B., Medley, I. and Harrison, G. (1999). Diagnostic stability of first-episode psychosis. Comparison of ICD-10 and DSM-III-R systems. *British Journal of Psychiatry*, **175**, 537–543.

Andreasen, N. C. and Flaum, M. (1995). The schizophrenia spectrum: perspectives from neuroimaging. In *Psychotic Continuum*, ed. A. Marneros, N. C. Andreasen and M. T. Tsuang. Berlin, Heidelberg, New York: Springer, pp. 91–106.

Angermeyer, M. C. and Klusmann, D. (1987). From social class to social stress: new developments in psychiatric epidemiology. In *From Social Class to Social Stress*, ed. M. C. Angermeyer. Berlin, Heidelberg, New York: Springer, pp. 1–14.

Angst, J. (1966). *Zur Ätiologie und Nosologie endogener depressiver Psychosen: eine genetische, soziologische und klinische Studie*. Berlin, Heidelberg, New York: Springer.

(1986). The course of schizoaffective disorders. In *Schizoaffective Psychoses*, ed. A. Marneros and M. T. Tsuang. Berlin: Springer, pp. 63–93.

(1995). Psychotic continuum or distinct entities: discussion. In *Psychotic Continuum*, ed. A. Marneros, N. C. Andreasen and M. T. Tsuang. Berlin, Heidelberg, New York: Springer, pp. 87–88.

Angst, J. and Clayton, P. (1986). Premorbid personality of depressive, bipolar, and schizophrenic patients with special reference to suicidal issues. *Comprehensive Psychiatry*, **27**, 511–532.

Angst, J. and Ernst, C. (1993). Current concepts of the classification of affective disorders. *International Clinical Psychopharmacology*, **8**, 211–215.

Angst, J. and Marneros, A. (2001). Bipolarity from ancient to modern times: conception, birth and rebirth. *Journal of Affective Disorders*, **67**, 3–19.

Angst, J. and Preisig, M. (1995). Course of a clinical cohort of unipolar, bipolar and schizoaffective patients. Results of a prospective study from 1959 to 1985. *Schweizer Archiv fur Neurologie und Psychiatrie*, **146**, 5–16.

Angst, J., Felder, W., Frey, R. and Stassen, H. H. (1978). The course of affective disorders. I. Change of diagnosis of monopolar, unipolar, and bipolar illness. *Archiv für Psychiatrie und Nervenkrankheiten*, **226**, 57–64.

Angst, J., Felder, W. and Lohmeyer, B. (1980). Course of schizoaffective psychoses: results of a follow-up study. *Schizophrenia Bulletin*, **6**, 579–585.

Angst, J., Stassen, H. H., Gross, G., Huber, G. and Stone, M. H. (1990). Suicide in affective and schizoaffective disorders. In *Affective and Schizoaffective Disorders*, ed. A. Marneros and M. T. Tsuang. Berlin, Heidelberg, New York: Springer, pp. 8–22.

APA (1987). *Diagnostic and Statistical Manual of Mental Disorders, 3rd edn, rev.* Washington, DC: American Psychiatric Association.

(1994). *Diagnostic and Statistical Manual of Mental Disorders, 4th edn.* Washington, DC: American Psychiatric Association.

(1997). American Psychiatric Association practice guideline for the treatment of patients with schizophrenia. *American Journal of Psychiatry*, **154** (Suppl. 4), 1–63.

Appia, O. (1964). *Evolution de la notion de bouffée déliriante polymorphe dans la psychiatrie française depuis Magnan jusqu'à nos jours (thesis)*. Paris: Sorbonne.

Aro, S., Aro, H., Salinto, M. and Keskimaki, I. (1995). Educational level and hospital use in mental disorders. A population-based study. *Acta Psychiatrica Scandinavica*, **91**, 305–312.

Asarnow, R. F. (1999). Neurocognitive impairments in schizophrenia: a piece of the epigenetic puzzle. *European Child and Adolescent Psychiatry*, **8** (Suppl. 1), 5–8.

Bardenstein, K. K. and McGlashan, T. H. (1990). Gender differences in affective, schizoaffective, and schizophrenic disorders. A review. *Schizophrenia Research*, **3**, 159–172.

Barry, H. and Barry, H. (1961). Season of birth. An epidemiological study in psychiatry. *Archives of General Psychiatry*, **5**, 292–300.

(1964). Season of birth in schizophrenics. *Archives of General Psychiatry*, **11**, 385–391.

Bassarath, L. (2001). Conduct disorder: a biopsychosocial review. *Canadian Journal of Psychiatry*, **46**, 609–616.

Beckmann, H. and Franzek, E. (2001). Cycloid psychoses and their differentiation from affective and schizophrenic psychoses. In *Contemporary Psychiatry*, ed. F. Henn, N. Sartorius, H. Helmchen and H. Lauter. Heidelberg: Springer. Volume 3, Part 1, pp. 387–398.

Beckmann, H., Fritze, J. and Lanczik, M. (1990). Prognostic validity of the cycloid psychoses. A prospective follow-up study. *Psychopathology*, **23**, 205–211.

Beckmann, H., Bartsch, A. J., Neumärker, K. J., Pfuhlmann, B., Verdaguer, M. F. and Franzek, E. (2000). Schizophrenias in the Wernicke–Kleist–Leonhard school. *American Journal of Psychiatry*, **157**, 1024–1025.

Beighley, P. S., Brown, G. R. and Thompson, J. W. (1992). DSM-III-R brief reactive psychosis among Air Force recruits. *Journal of Clinical Psychiatry*, **53**, 283–288.

Benes, F. M. (1995). Microscopic findings in the cortex and hippocampus of schizophrenic and schizoaffective patients. In *Psychotic Continuum*, ed. A. Marneros, N. C. Andreasen and M. T. Tsuang. Berlin, Heidelberg, New York: Springer, pp. 127–136.

Berger, J., Scheurer, H., Honecker, Y., Andritsch, F. and Six, A. T. (1999). Straffällige Alkohol- und Drogenabhängige. Identifikation prognostisch günstiger und ungünstiger Patientengruppen im Massregelvollzug nach § 64 StGB. *Fortschritte der Neurologie-Psychiatrie*, **67**, 502–508.

Berrios, G. E. and Beer, D. (1994). The notion of a unitary psychosis: a conceptual history. *History of Psychiatry*, **5**, 13–36.

Biehl, H., Maurer, K., Jablensky, A., Cooper, J. E. and Tomov, T. (1989a). The WHO Psychological Impairments Rating Schedule (WHO/PIRS). I. Introducing a new instrument for rating observed behaviour and the rationale of the psychological impairment concept. *British Journal of Psychiatry* (Suppl. 7), 68–70.

Biehl, H., Maurer, K., Jung, E. and Krumm, B. (1989b). The WHO Psychological Impairments Rating Schedule (WHO/PIRS). II. Impairments in Schizophrenics in cross-sectional and longitudinal perspective – the Mannheim experience in two independent samples. *British Journal of Psychiatry* (Suppl. 7), 71–77.

Binswanger, O. (1928). Die klinische Stellung der Degenerationspsychosen. *Archiv für Psychiatrie und Nervenkrankheiten*, **83**, 299–375.

Birnbaum, K. (1923). *Der Aufbau der Psychose*. Berlin: Springer.

Bleich, A. and Moskowits, L. (2000). Post-traumatic stress disorder with psychotic features. *Croatian Medical Journal*, **41**, 442–445.

Bleuler, E. (1911). *Dementia praecox oder Gruppe der Schizophrenien*. Leipzig, Wien: Deuticke.

Bleuler, M. (1972). *Die schizophrenen Geistesstörungen im Lichte langjähriger Kranken- und Familiengeschichten*. Stuttgart: Thieme.

Blöink, R., Brieger, P., Akiskal, H. S. and Marneros, A. (2004). Reliability and validity of the TEMPS-A scale on the basis of the NEO-FFI questionnaire. *Journal of Affective Disorders*: in press.

Boeters, V. (1971). *Die oneiroiden Emotionspsychosen*. Basel: Karger.

Bonhoeffer, K. (1907). *Klinische Beiträge zur Lehre von den Degenerationspsychosen*. Halle: Marhold.

Borkenau, P. and Ostendorf, F. (1993). *NEO-Fünf-Faktoren Inventar (NEO-FFI)*. Göttingen, Bern, Toronto, Seattle: Hogrefe.

Bottlender, R., Jäger, M., Strauss, A. and Möller, H. J. (2000). Suicidality in bipolar compared to unipolar depressed inpatients. *European Archives of Psychiatry and Clinical Neuroscience*, **250**, 257–261.

Bradbury, T. N. and Miller, G. A. (1985). Season of birth in schizophrenia: a review of evidence, methodology, and etiology. *Psychological Bulletin*, **98**, 569–594.

Bräunig, P. and Fimmers, R. (1995). Long-term course and outcome of cycloid psychoses in comparison to schizoaffective psychoses. In *Leonhard's Impact on Modern Psychiatry*, ed. H. Beckmann and K.-J. Neumärker. Berlin, Wiesbaden: Ullstein Mosby, pp. 69–75.

Brewin, J., Cantwell, R., Dalkin, T. *et al.* (1997). Incidence of schizophrenia in Nottingham. A comparison of two cohorts, 1978–80 and 1992–94. *British Journal of Psychiatry*, **171**, 140–144.

Brieger, P., Blöink, R., Sommer, S. and Marneros, A. (2001). Affective symptoms at index hospitalization in childhood and depressive symptoms in adulthood: a 'catch-up' study. *Journal of Affective Disorders*, **66**, 263–266.

Brockington, I. F., Perris, C., Kendell, R. E., Hillier, V. E. and Wainwright, S. (1982a). The course and outcome of cycloid psychosis. *Psychological Medicine*, **12**, 97–105.

Brockington, I. F., Perris, C. and Meltzer, H. Y. (1982b). Cycloid psychoses. Diagnosis and heuristic value. *Journal of Nervous and Mental Disease*, 651–656.

Buda, M. and Tsuang, M. T. (1990). The epidemiology of suicide: implications for clinical practice. In *Suicide over the Life Cycle*, ed. S. J. Blumenthal and D. J. Kupfer. Washington, London: American Psychiatric Press, pp. 17–96.

Bulik, C. M., Prescott, C. A. and Kendler, K. S. (2001). Features of childhood sexual abuse and the development of psychiatric and substance use disorders. *British Journal of Psychiatry*, **179**, 444–449.

Calabrese, J. R., Rapport, D. J., Findling, R. L., Shelton, M. D. and Kimmel, S. (2000). Rapid-cycling bipolar disorder. In *Bipolar Disorders. 100 Years After Manic-depressive Insanity*, ed. A. Marneros and J. Angst. Dordrecht, Boston, London: Kluwer.

Campbell, M. and Malone, R. P. (1991). Mental retardation and psychiatric disorders. *Hospital and Community Psychiatry*, **42**, 374–379.

Carpenter, W. T., Buchanan, R. W. and Kirkpatrick, B. (1995). Schizophrenia: disease entity, disease entities, or domains of psychopathology. In *Psychotic Continuum*, ed. A. Marneros, N. C. Andreasen and M. T. Tsuang. Berlin, Heidelberg, New York: Springer, pp. 137–149.

Cerrolaza, M. and Cleghorn, R. A. (1971). Atypical psychoses. A search for certainty in this ambiguous borderland. *Canadian Psychiatric Association Journal*, **16**, 507–514.

Chiniwala, M., Alfonso, C. A., Torres, J. R. and Lefer, J. (1996). Koro in an immigrant from Guinea with brief psychotic disorder [letter to the editor]. *American Journal of Psychiatry*, **153**, 736.

Ciompi, L. and Müller, C. (1976). *Lebensweg und Alter der Schizophrenen. Eine katamnestische Langzeitstudie bis ins Senium*. Berlin, Heidelberg, New York: Springer.

Clark, J. A. and Mallett, B. L. (1963). A follow-up study of schizophrenia and depression in young adults. *British Journal of Psychiatry*, **109**, 491–499.

Collins, P. Y., Wig, N. N., Day, R. *et al.* (1996). Psychosocial and biological aspects of acute brief psychoses in three developing country sites. *Psychiatric Quarterly*, **67**, 177–193.

Collins, P. Y., Varma, V. K., Wig, N. N., Mojtabai, R., Day, R. and Susser, E. (1999). Fever and acute brief psychosis in urban and rural settings in north India. *British Journal of Psychiatry*, **174**, 520–524.

Collomb, H. (1965). Bouffée délirante en psychiatrie africaine. *Psychopathologie Africaine*, **1**, 167–239.

Constant, J. (1972). Les bouffées délirantes an Guadeloupe: essai d'analyse sémiologique, psychologique et culturelle à propos de 112 observations. *Psychopathologie Africaine*, **8**, 169–199.

Cooper, J. and Sartorius, N. (1977). Cultural and temporal variations in schizophrenia: a speculation on the importance of industrialization. *British Journal of Psychiatry*, **130**, 50–55.

Cooper, J. E., Jablensky, A. and Sartorius, N. (1990). WHO collaborative studies on acute psychoses using the SCAAPS schedule. In *Psychiatry: A World Perspective: Proceedings of the VIII World Congress of Psychiatry, Athens*, ed. C. N. Stefanis, A. D. Rabavilas and C. R. Soldatos. *12–19 October 1989, Vol. I*. New York: Elsevier, pp. 185–192.

Copolov, D. L., McGorry, P. D., Singh, B. S., Proeve, M. and Van Riel, R. (1990). The influence of gender on the classification of psychotic disorders – a multidiagnostic approach. *Acta Psychiatrica Scandinavica*, **82**, 8–13.

Cornblatt, B. A., Lencz, T. and Kane, J. M. (2001). Treatment of the schizophrenia prodrome: is it presently ethical? *Schizophrenia Research*, **51**, 31–38.

Coryell, W. and Winokur, G. (1980). Diagnosis, family, and follow-up studies. In *Mania. An Evolving Concept*, ed. R. H. Belmaker and H. M. van Praag. Jamaica, NY: Spectrum.

Costa, P. T. and McCrae, R. R. (1992). *Revised NEO Personality Inventory (NEO PI-R) and NEO Five-Factor Inventory (NEO-FFI)*. Odessa, FL: Psychological Assessment Resources.

Crow, T. J. (1980). Molecular pathology of schizophrenia: more than one disease process? *British Medical Journal*, **280**, 66–68.

(1995). Psychotic continuum or disease entities? The critical impact of nosology on the problem of aetiology. In *Psychotic Continuum*, ed. A. Marneros, N. C. Andreasen and M. T. Tsuang. Berlin, Heidelberg, New York: Springer, pp. 151–163.

(2000). Bipolar shifts as disorders of the bi-hemispheric integration of language: implications for the genetic origins of the psychotic continuum. In *Bipolar Disorders. 100 Years After Manic-depressive Insanity*, ed. A. Marneros and J. Angst. Dordrecht, Boston, London: Kluwer.

Cuesta, M. J., Peralta, V. and Caro, F. (1999). Premorbid personality in psychoses. *Schizophrenia Bulletin*, **25**, 801–811.

Cutting, J. C., Clare, A. W. and Mann, A. H. (1978). Cycloid psychosis: an investigation of the diagnostic concept. *Psychological Medicine*, **8**, 637–648.

Dahl, A. A. (1986). The DSM-III classification of the functional psychoses and the Norwegian tradition. *Acta Psychiatrica Scandinavica* (Suppl.) **328**, 45–53.

Dahl, A. A., Cloninger, C. R., Guze, S. B. and Retterstol, N. (1992). Convergence of American and Scandinavian diagnoses of functional psychoses. *Comprehensive Psychiatry*, **33**, 13–16.

Dalkin, T., Murphy, P., Glazebrook, C., Medley, I. and Harrison, G. (1994). Premorbid personality in first-onset psychosis. *British Journal of Psychiatry*, **164**, 202–207.

Das, S. K., Malhotra, S. and Basu, D. (1999). Family study of acute and transient psychotic disorders: comparison with schizophrenia. *Social Psychiatry and Psychiatric Epidemiology*, **34**, 328–332.

Das, S. K., Malhotra, S., Basu, D. and Malhotra, R. (2001). Testing the stress-vulnerability hypothesis in ICD-10-diagnosed acute and transient psychotic disorders. *Acta Psychiatrica Scandinavica*, **104**, 56–58.

Davidson, L. and McGlashan, T. H. (1997). The varied outcomes of schizophrenia. *Canadian Journal of Psychiatry*, **42**, 34–43.

Devillières, P., Opitz, M., Clervoy, P. and Stephany, J. (1996). Bouffée délirante et privation de sommeil. *Encéphale*, **22**, 229–231.

Dietrich, D. E., Gödecke-Koch, T., Richter-Witte, C. and Emrich, H. M. (2004). Lamotrigine in the treatment of confusion psychosis. *Pharmacopsychiatry (in press)*.

Dohrenwend, B. P. and Dohrenwend, B. S. (1976). Sex differences and psychiatric disorders. *American Journal of Sociology*, **81**, 1447–1454.

Dohrenwend, B. P., Levav, I., Shrout, P. E. *et al.* (1992). Socioeconomic status and psychiatric disorders: the causation–selection issue. *Science*, **255**, 946–952.

  (1998). Ethnicity, socioeconomic status, and psychiatric disorders: a test of the social causation–social selection issue. In *Adversity, Stress, and Psychopathology*, ed. B. P. Dohrenwend. New York: Oxford University Press, pp. 283–318.

Drake, R. E., Gates, C., Whitaker, A. and Cotton, P. G. (1985). Suicide among schizophrenics: a review. *Comprehensive Psychiatry*, **26**, 90–100.

Duffy, A. and Grof, P. (2001). Psychiatric diagnoses in the context of genetic studies of bipolar disorder. *Bipolar Disorders*, **3**, 270–275.

Dunham, H. W. (1965). *Community and Schizophrenia*. Detroit: Wayne State University Press.

Eaton, W. W. (1975). Marital status and schizophrenia. *Acta Psychiatrica Scandinavica*, **52**, 320–329.

  (1985). Epidemiology of schizophrenia. *Epidemiologic Reviews*, **7**, 105–126.

Ellison, Z., van Os, J. and Murray, R. (1998). Special feature: childhood personality characteristics of schizophrenia: manifestations of, or risk factors for, the disorder? *Journal of Personality Disorders*, **12**, 247–261.

Endicott, J., Spitzer, R. L., Fleiss, J. L. and Cohen, J. (1976). The global assessment scale. A procedure for measuring overall severity of psychiatric disturbance. *Archives of General Psychiatry*, **33**, 766–771.

Ey, H. (1952). Grundlagen einer organo-dynamischen Auffassung der Psychiatrie. *Fortschritte der Neurologie-Psychiatrie*, **20**, 195–209.

  (1954). 'Bouffées délirantes' et psychoses hallucinatoires aigus. *Études psychiatriques. Vol. 3: Structure des psychoses aigues et déstructuration de la conscience*. Paris: Desclée de Brouwer, pp. 203–324.

Faraone, S. V., Tsuang, M. T. and Tsuang, D. W. (1999). *Genetics of Mental Disorders*. New York, London: Guilford Press.

Fekkes, D., Pepplinkhuizen, L., Verheij, R. and Bruinvels, J. (1994). Abnormal plasma levels of serine, methionine, and taurine in transient acute polymorphic psychosis. *Psychiatry Research*, **51**, 11–18.

Ferrey, G. and Zebdi, S. (1999). Evolution et pronostic des troubles psychotiques aigus (bouffée délirante polymorphe). *Encéphale*, **25**, Spec No 3, 26–32.

Fish, F. (1964). The cycloid psychoses. *Comprehensive Psychiatry*, **5**, 155–169.

Franzek, E. and Beckmann, H. (1992). Season-of-birth effect reveals the existence of etiologically different groups of schizophrenia. *Biological Psychiatry*, **32**, 375–378.

   (1998a). Different genetic background of schizophrenia spectrum psychoses: a twin study. *American Journal of Psychiatry*, **155**, 76–83.

   (1998b). *Psychosen des schizophrenen Spektrums bei Zwillingen*. Berlin: Springer.

Franzek, E., Becker, T., Hofmann, E., Flohl, W., Stöber, G. and Beckmann, H. (1996). Is computerized tomography ventricular abnormality related to cycloid psychosis? *Biological Psychiatry*, **40**, 1255–1266.

Fritsch, W. (1975). Die prämorbide Persönlichkeit der Schizophrenen in der Literatur der letzten 100 Jahre. *Fortschritte der Neurologie-Psychiatrie*, **44**, 323–372.

Fukuda, T. (1990). Cycloid psychoses as atypical psychoses: 'concordance' and 'discordance'. *Psychopathology*, **23**, 253–258.

Gaebel, W., Janner, M., Frommann, N. *et al.* (2002). First vs. multiple episode schizophrenia: two-year outcome of intermittent and maintenance medication strategies. *Schizophrenia Research*, **53**, 145–159.

German, G. A. (1972). Aspects of clinical psychiatry in sub-Saharan Africa. *British Journal of Psychiatry*, **121**, 461–479.

Gmur, M. and Tschopp, A. (1987). Die Broken-home-Häufigkeit bei Schizophrenen. Eine Untersuchung an 239 sozialpsychiatrisch behandelten Patienten. *Sozial- und Präventivmedizin*, **32**, 157–160.

Goldberg, E. M. and Morrison, S. L. (1963). Schizophrenia and social class. *British Journal of Psychiatry*, **109**, 785–802.

Goldman, H. H., Skodol, A. E. and Lave, T. R. (1992). Revising axis V for DSM-IV: a review of measures of social functioning. *American Journal of Psychiatry*, **149**, 1148–1156.

Goldney, R. D. (1981). Parental loss and reported childhood stress in young women who attempt suicide. *Acta Psychiatrica Scandinavica*, **64**, 34–47.

Goldstein, M. J. (1990). Psychosocial factors relating to etiology and course of schizophrenia. In *Handbook of Schizophrenia, Vol. 4*, ed. H. A. Nasrallah. Amsterdam, New York, Oxford: Elsevier.

Goodwin, F. K. and Jamison, K. R., eds. (1990). *Manic-depressive Illness*. New York, Oxford: Oxford University Press.

Grossman, L. S., Harrow, M., Fudala, J. L. and Meltzer, H. Y. (1984). The longitudinal course of schizoaffective disorders. A prospective follow-up study. *Journal of Nervous and Mental Disease*, **172**, 140–149.

Gupta, S., Black, D. W., Arndt, S., Hubbard, W. C. and Andreasen, N. C. (1998). Factors associated with suicide attempts among patients with schizophrenia. *Psychiatric Services*, **49**, 1353–1355.

Gurrera, R. J., Nestor, P. G. and O'Donnell, B. F. (2000). Personality traits in schizophrenia: comparison with a community sample. *Journal of Nervous and Mental Disease*, **188**, 31–35.

Häfner, H. (1987). Epidemiology of schizphrenia. In *Search for the Causes of Schizophrenia*, ed. H. Häfner, W. F. Gattaz and W. Janzarik. Berlin, Heidelberg, New York: Springer.

Häfner, H. and an der Heiden, W. (1997). Epidemiology of schizophrenia. *Canadian Journal of Psychiatry*, **42**, 139–151.

Häfner, H., Riecher, A., Maurer, K., Löffler, W., Munk-Jørgensen, P. and Strömgren, E. (1989). How does gender influence age at first hospitalization for schizophrenia? A transnational case register study. *Psychological Medicine*, **19**, 903–918.

Häfner, H., Maurer, K., Löffler, W. and Riecher-Rössler, A. (1991). Schizophrenie und Lebensalter. *Nervenarzt*, **62**, 536–548.

Häfner, H., an der Heiden, W., Behrens, S. *et al.* (1998). Causes and consequences of the gender difference in age at onset of schizophrenia. *Schizophrenia Bulletin*, **24**, 99–113.

Harrison, G., Gunnell, D., Glazebrook, C., Page, K. and Kwiecinski, R. (2001). Association between schizophrenia and social inequality at birth: case-control study. *British Journal of Psychiatry*, **179**, 346–350.

Harrison, G., Owens, D., Holton, A., Neilson, D. and Boot, D. (1988). A prospective study of severe mental disorders in Afro-Caribbean patients. *Psychological Medicine*, **18**, 643–658.

Hatotani, N. (1983). Nosological consideration of periodic psychoses. In *Neurobiology of Periodic Psychoses*, ed. N. Hatotani and J. Nomura. Tokyo: IgaKu-Shoin, pp. 1–14.

(1996). The concept of 'atypical psychoses': special reference to its development in Japan. *Psychiatry and Clinical Neurosciences*, **50**, 1–10.

Hatotani, N. and Nomura, J. (1983). *Neurobiology of Periodic Psychoses*. Tokyo: IgaKu-Shoin.

Hawton, K. and Van Heeringen, K., eds. (2000). *The International Handbook of Suicide and Attempted Suicide*. Chichester: Wiley.

Hecht, H., van Calker, D., Spraul, G. *et al.* (1997). Premorbid personality in patients with uni- and bipolar affective disorders and controls: assessment by the Biographical Personality Interview (BPI). *European Archives of Psychiatry and Clinical Neuroscience*, **247**, 23–30.

Heikkinen, M., Isometsa, E. T., Henriksson, M. M., Marttunen, M. J., Aro, H. M. and Lonnqvist, J. K. (1997). Psychosocial factors and completed suicide in personality disorders. *Acta Psychiatrica Scandinavica*, **95**, 49–57.

Hoch, A. and MacCurdy, J. T. (1921). *Benign Stupors; A Study of a New Manic-depressive Reaction Type*. New York: The Macmillan Company.

Höffler, J., Bräunig, P., Krüger, S. and Ludvik, M. (1997). Morphology according to cranial computed tomography of first-episode cycloid psychosis and its long-term-course: differences compared to schizophrenia. *Acta Psychiatrica Scandinavica*, **96**, 184–187.

Hollingshead, A. B. and Redlich, F. C. (1958). *Social Class and Mental Illness*. New York: Wiley.

Hopper, K. and Wanderling, J. (2000). Revisiting the developed versus developing country distinction in course and outcome in schizophrenia: results from ISoS, the WHO collaborative followup project. International Study of Schizophrenia. *Schizophrenia Bulletin*, **26**, 835–846.

Horgan, D. (1981). Changes of diagnosis to manic-depressive illness. *Psychological Medicine*, **11**, 517–523.

Huber, G. (1957). *Pneumencephalographische und psychopathologische Bilder bei endogenen Psychosen*. Berlin, Göttingen, Heidelberg: Springer.

Huber, G., Gross, G. and Schüttler, R. (1979). *Schizophrenie. Eine verlaufs- und sozialpsychiatrische Langzeitstudie.* Berlin: Springer.

Hunt, R. C. and Appel, K. E. (1936). Prognosis in the psychoses lying midway between schizophrenia and manic-depressive psychoses. *American Journal of Psychiatry,* **93,** 313–339.

INSERM (1969). Classification française des troubles mentau. *Bulletin de l'Institut National de la Santé et de la Recherche Médicale,* **24,** 1–29.

Inui, K., Motomura, E., Okushima, R., Kaige, H., Inoue, K. and Nomura, J. (1998). Electroencephalographic findings in patients with DSM-IV mood disorder, schizophrenia, and other psychotic disorders. *Biological Psychiatry,* **43,** 69–75.

Isohanni, I., Jarvelin, M. R., Nieminen, P. *et al.* (1998). School performance as a predictor of psychiatric hospitalization in adult life. A 28-year follow-up in the Northern Finland 1966 Birth Cohort. *Psychological Medicine,* **28,** 967–974.

Ivezic, S., Bagaric, A., Oruc, L., Mimica, N. and Ljubin, T. (2000). Psychotic symptoms and comorbid psychiatric disorders in Croatian combat-related posttraumatic stress disorder patients. *Croatian Medical Journal,* **41,** 179–183.

Iwawaki, A., Fujiya, K. and Kobayashi, K. (1996). Acute polymorphic psychosis in adults with mild intellectual deficits. *Psychiatry and Clinical Neurosciences,* **50,** 109–113.

Jablensky, A., Sartorius, N., Ernberg, G. *et al.* (1992). Schizophrenia: manifestations, incidence and course in different cultures. A World Health Organization ten-country study. *Psychological Medicine. Monograph Suppl.,* **20,** 1–97.

Jablensky, A., Schwarz, R. and Tomov, T. (1980). WHO collaborative study on impairments and disabilities associated with schizophrenic disorders. A preliminary communication: objectives and methods. *Acta Psychiatrica Scandinavica* (Suppl.) **62,** 152–163.

Janakiramaiah, N., Gangadhar, B. N., Pandit, L. V., Ravi, V., Desai, A. and Subbakrishna, D. K. (1998). Viral infection in drug-naive, DSM-IV brief psychotic disorder patients. *Biological Psychiatry,* **43** (Suppl. 8), 43S-43S.

Janzarik, W. (1968). *Schizophrene Verläufe. Eine strukturdynamische Interpretation.* Berlin, Heidelberg, New York: Springer.

Jaspers, K. (1913). *Allgemeine Psychopathologie.* Berlin: Springer.

Jauch, D. A. and Carpenter, W. T. (1988a). Reactive psychosis: I. Does the pre-DSM-III concept define a third psychosis? *Journal of Nervous and Mental Disease,* **176,** 72–81.

(1988b). Reactive psychosis: II. Does DSM-III-R define a third psychosis? *Journal of Nervous and Mental Disease,* **176,** 82–86.

Jilek, W. G. and Jilek-Aall, L. (1970). Transient psychoses in Africans. *Psychiatria Clinica,* **3,** 337–364.

Johnson-Sabine, E. C., Mann, A. H., Jacoby, R. J. *et al.* (1983). Bouffée délirante: an examination of its current status. *Psychological Medicine,* **13,** 771–778.

Jones, P. B., Bebbington, P., Foerster, A. *et al.* (1993). Premorbid social underachievement in schizophrenia. Results from the Camberwell Collaborative Psychosis Study. *British Journal of Psychiatry,* **162,** 65–71.

Jones, P., Rodgers, B., Murray, R. and Marmot, M. (1994). Child development risk factors for adult schizophrenia in the British 1946 birth cohort. *Lancet,* **344,** 1398–1402.

Jönsson, S. A. T. (1991). Marriage rate and fertility in cycloid psychosis: comparison with affective disorder, schizophrenia and the general population. *European Archives of Psychiatry and Clinical Neuroscience*, **241**, 119–125.

(1995). Zykloide Psychose: die unterschiedlichen Einflüsse der Symptome. In *Emotionspsychopathologie und zykloide Psychosen*, ed. P. Bräunig. Stuttgart, New York: Schattauer, pp. 183–189.

Jönsson, S. A. T., Jonsson, H., Nyman, A. K. and Nyman, G. E. (1991a). The concept of cycloid psychosis: sensitivity and specifity of syndromes derived by multivariate clustering techniques. *Acta Psychiatrica Scandinavica*, **83**, 353–362.

Jönsson, S. A. T., Jönsson, H. and Nyman, G. E. (1991b). The concept of cycloid psychosis: the discriminatory power of symptoms. *Acta Psychiatrica Scandinavica*, **84**, 22–25.

Jørgensen, P. (1994a). Course and outcome in delusional beliefs. *Psychopathology*, **27**, 89–99.

(1994b). Course and outcome in delusional disorders. *Psychopathology*, **27**, 79–88.

(1995). Comparative outcome of first-admission patients with delusional beliefs. *European Psychiatry*, **10**, 276–281.

Jørgensen, P. and Jensen, J. (1994a). Delusional beliefs in first admitters. A clinical description. *Psychopathology*, **27**, 100–112.

(1994b). How to understand the formation of delusional beliefs: a proposal. *Psychopathology*, **27**, 64–72.

(1994c). What predicts the persistence of delusional beliefs? *Psychopathology*, **27**, 73–78.

Jørgensen, P., Bennedsen, B., Christensen, J. and Hyllested, A. (1996). Acute and transient psychotic disorder: comorbidity with personality disorder. *Acta Psychiatrica Scandinavica*, **94**, 460–464.

(1997). Acute and transient psychotic disorder: a 1-year follow-up study. *Acta Psychiatrica Scandinavica*, **96**, 150–154.

Jung, E., Krumm, B., Biehl, H., Maurer, K. and Bauer-Schubart, C. (1989). *Mannheimer Skala zur Einschätzung sozialer Behinderung, DAS-M*. Weinheim: Beltz.

Kahlbaum, L. (1863). *Die Gruppirung psychischer Krankheiten und die Eintheilung der Seelenstörungen*. Danzig: Kafemann.

(1884). Über cyclisches Irresein. *Allgemeine Zeitschrift für Psychiatrie*, **40**, 405–406.

Kasanin, J. (1933). The acute schizoaffective psychoses. *American Journal of Psychiatry*, **13**, 97–126.

Kay, S. R., Opler, L. A. and Lindenmayer, J. P. (1989). The Positive and Negative Syndrome Scale (PANSS): rationale and standardisation. *British Journal of Psychiatry* (Suppl. 7), 59–67.

Kendler, K. S. and Walsh, D. (1995). Schizophreniform disorder, delusional disorder and psychotic disorder not otherwise specified: clinical features, outcome and familial psychopathology. *Acta Psychiatrica Scandinavica*, **91**, 370–378.

Kendler, K. S., McGuire, M., Gruenberg, A. M., O'Hare, A., Spellman, M. and Walsh, D. (1993a). The Roscommon Family Study. I. methods, diagnosis of probands and risk of schizophrenia in relatives. *Archives of General Psychiatry*, **50**, 527–540.

Kendler, K. S., McGuire, M., Gruenberg, A. M., Spellman, M., O'Hare, A. and Walsh, D. (1993b). The Roscommon Family Study. II. The risk of nonschizophrenic nonaffective psychoses in relatives. *Archives of General Psychiatry*, **50**, 645–652.

Kentros, M., Smith, T. E., Hull, J., McKee, M., Terkelsen, K. and Capalbo, C. (1997). Stability of personality traits in schizophrenia and schizoaffective disorder: a pilot project. *Journal of Nervous and Mental Disease*, **185**, 549–555.

Kimura, S., Fujito, T. and Wakabayashi, T. (1980). A contribution to the course and prognosis of the atypical psychosis. *Folia Psychiatrica et Neurologica Japonica*, **34**, 419–432.

Kimura, S., Ohya, D., Koh, T. and Iwamura, H. (1984). Course and prognosis of endogenous-phasic psychoses in adolescence. *Psychopathology*, **17**, 137–143.

Kirby, G. H. (1913). The catatonic syndrome and its relation to manic-depressive insanity. *Journal of Nervous and Mental Disease*, **40**, 694–704.

Kirov, K. (1972). Untersuchungen über den Verlauf zykloider Psychosen. *Psychiatrie, Neurologie und Medizinische Psychologie*, **24**, 726–732.

Kleining, G. and Moore, H. (1975a). Soziale Mobilität in der Bundesrepublik Deutschland – I. Klassenmobilität. *Kölner Zeitschrift für Soziologie und Sozialpsychologie*, **27**, 273–292.

Kleining, G. and Moore, H. (1975b). Soziale Mobilität in der Bundesrepublik Deutschland – II. Status-oder Prestigemobilität. *Kölner Zeitschrift für Soziologie und Sozialpsychologie*, **27**, 502–552.

Kleist, K. (1924). Über die gegenwärtigen Strömungen in der klinischen Psychiatrie. *Allgemeine Zeitschrift für Psychiatrie*, **81**, 389–393.

(1925). Über die gegenwärtigen Strömungen in der klinischen Psychiatrie. Referat Naturf.-Vers. Innsbruck 1924. *Allgemeine Zeitschrift für Psychiatrie*, **82**, 1–41.

(1926). Über cycloide Degenerationspsychosen, besonders Verwirrtheits- und Motilitäts-psychosen. *Zentralblatt für die gesamte Neurologie und Psychiatrie*, **44**, 655–657.

(1928). Über cycloide, paranoide und epileptoide Psychosen und über die Frage der Degenerationspsychosen. *Schweizer Archiv fur Neurologie, Neurochirurgie und Psychiatrie*, **23**, 3–37.

(1953). Die Gliederung der neuropsychischen Erkrankungen. *Monatsschrift für Psychiatrie und Neurologie*, **125**, 526–554.

Koehler, K. (1983). Prognostic prediction in RDC schizo-affective disorder on the basis of first-rank symptoms weighted in terms of outcome. *Psychiatria Clinica*, **16**, 186–197.

Kraepelin, E. (1893). *Psychiatrie: ein kurzes Lehrbuch für Studirende und Ärzte, 4., vollst. umgearb. Aufl.* Leipzig: Abel.

(1896). *Psychiatrie: ein Lehrbuch für Studirende und Ärzte, 5., vollständig umgearb. Aufl.* Leipzig: J. A. Barth.

(1899). *Psychiatrie: ein Lehrbuch für Studirende und Ärzte, 6., vollst. umgearb. Aufl.* Leipzig: J. A. Barth.

(1899/1990). *Psychiatry: A Textbook for Students and Physicians (Translation of the 6th edition of: Psychiatrie. Ein Lehrbuch für Studirende und Ärzte).* ed. J. M. Quen. Canton, MA: Science History Publications/USA.

(1920). Die Erscheinungsformen des Irreseins. *Zeitschrift für die gesamte Neurologie und Psychiatrie*, **62**, 1–29.

Kronmüller, K. T. and Mundt, C. (1999). Interaktionsmuster. In *Handbuch der unipolaren und bipolaren Erkrankungen*, ed. A. Marneros. Stuttgart: Thieme, pp. 390–431.

Kunugi, H., Nanko, S. and Murray, R. M. (2001). Obstetric complications and schizophrenia: prenatal underdevelopment and subsequent neurodevelopmental impairment. *British Journal of Psychiatry*, **178**, S25–29.

Kurosawa, R. (1961). Untersuchung der atypischen endogenen Psychosen (periodische Psychosen). *Psychiatrie, Neurologie und Medizinische Psychologie*, **13**, 364–370.

Labhardt, F. (1963). *Die schizophrenieähnlichen Emotionspsychosen*. Berlin: Springer.

Lanczik, M., Fritze, J. and Beckmann, H. (1990). Puerperal and cycloid psychoses: results of a retrospective study. *Psychopathology*, **23**, 220–227.

Landis, J. R. and Koch, G. G. (1977). The measurement of observer agreement for categorical data. *Biometrics*, **33**, 159–174.

Langfeldt, G. (1939). *The Schizophreniform States*. Kopenhagen: Munksgaard.

Lazaratou, H., Dellatolas, G., Moreau, T. and Chaigneau, H. (1989). Bouffée délirante et évolution schizophrénique: rôle pronostique de la classification DSM III. *Psychiatry and Psychobiology*, **3**, 297–304.

Lee, A. S. and Murray, R. M. (1988). The long-term outcome of Maudsley depressives. *British Journal of Psychiatry*, **153**, 741–751.

Legrain, M. (1886). *Du délire chez les dégénérés*. Paris: Delahaye/Lescrosnier [reprint 1978 Nendeln/Liechtenstein: Kraus].

Leibrand, W. and Wettley, A. (1961). *Der Wahnsinn. Geschichte der abendländischen Psychopathologie*. Freiburg, München: Karl Alber.

Leonhard, K. (1934). Atypische endogene Psychosen im Lichte der Familienforschung. *Zeitschrift für die gesamte Neurologie und Psychiatrie*, **149**, 520–562.

(1939). Fragen der Erbbegutachtung bei den atypischen Psychosen. *Allgemeine Zeitschrift für Psychiatrie*, **112**, 391.

(1957). *Die Aufteilung der endogenen Psychosen. 1. Auflage*. Berlin: Akademie-Verlag.

(1961). Cycloid psychoses – endogenous psychoses which are neither schizophrenic nor manic-depressive. *Journal of Mental Science*, **107**, 633–648.

(1983). Is the concept of 'schizo-affective psychoses' prognostically of value? *Psychiatria Clinica*, **16**, 178–185.

(1995). *Die Aufteilung der endogenen Psychosen und ihre differenzierte Ätiologie. 7., neubearbeitete und ergänzte Auflage*. Stuttgart: Thieme.

(1999). *Classification of Endogenous Psychoses and their Differential Etiology (2nd rev. and enlarged edn., ed. H. Beckmann)*. Wien, New York: Springer.

Leung, A. and Chue, P. (2000). Sex differences in schizophrenia, a review of the literature. *Acta Psychiatrica Scandinavica* (Suppl.) **401**, 3–38.

Lewine, R. R. J. (1988). Gender and schizophrenia. In *Handbook of Schizophrenia. Vol. 3: Nosology, Epidemiology and Genetics of Schizophrenia*, ed. H. A. Nasrallah. Amsterdam, New York, Oxford: Elsevier.

Lewis, N. D. C. and Pietrowski, Z. A. (1954). Clinical diagnosis of manic-depressive psychosis. *Proceedings of the Annual Meeting of the American Psychopathological Association*, **44**, 25–38.

Lindvall, M., Axelsson, R. and Öhman, R. (1993). Incidence of cycloid psychosis. A clinical study of first-admission psychotic patients. *European Archives of Psychiatry and Clinical Neuroscience*, **242**, 197–202.

Littlewood, R. and Lipsedge, M. (1981). Acute psychotic reactions in Caribbean-born patients. *Psychological Medicine*, **11**, 303–318.

Loranger, A. W. (1984). Sex difference in age at onset of schizophrenia. *Archives of General Psychiatry*, **41**, 157–161.

Lysaker, P. H., Meyer, P. S., Evans, J. D., Clements, C. A. and Marks, K. A. (2001). Childhood sexual trauma and psychosocial functioning in adults with schizophrenia. *Psychiatric Services*, **52**, 1485–1488.

Magnan, V. (1893). *Leçons cliniques sur les maladies mentales. 2. Aufl.* Paris: Battaille.

Magnan, V. and Legrain, M. (1895). *Les dégénérés. Etat mental et syndromes épisodiques.* Paris: Rueff.

Maj, M. (1984). The evolution of some European diagnostic concepts relevant to the category of schizoaffective psychoses. *Psychopathology*, **17**, 158–167.

(1988). Clinical course and outcome of cycloid psychotic disorders: a three-year prospective study. *Acta Psychiatrica Scandinavica*, **78**, 182–187.

(1989). A family study of two subgroups of schizoaffective patients. *British Journal of Psychiatry*, **154**, 640–643.

(1990a). Cycloid psychotic disorder: validation of the concept by means of a follow-up and a family study. *Psychopathology*, **23**, 196–204.

(1990b). Mobidity risk for major psychiatric disorders in first-degree relatives of two subgroups of schizoaffective patients. In *Psychiatry: A World Perspective: Proceedings of the VIII World Congress of Psychiatry, Athens,* ed. C. N. Stefanis, A. D. Rabavilas and C. R. Soldatos, *12–19 October 1989, Vol. I.* New York: Elsevier, pp. 394–399.

Malhotra, S., Varma, V. K., Misra, A. K., Das, S., Wig, N. N. and Santosh, P. J. (1998). Onset of acute psychotic states in India: a study of sociodemographic, seasonal and biological factors. *Acta Psychiatrica Scandinavica*, **97**, 125–131.

Mall, G. (1952). Beitrag zur Gjessingschen Thyroxinbehandlung der periodischen Katatonien. *Archiv für Psychiatrie und Zeitschrift für Neurologie*, **187**, 381–403.

Manschreck, T. C. and Petri, M. (1978). The atypical psychoses. *Culture, Medicine and Psychiatry*, **2**, 233–268.

Manton, K. G., Korten, A., Woodbury, M. A., Anker, M. and Jablensky, A. (1994). Symptom profiles of psychiatric disorders based on graded disease classes: an illustration using data from the WHO International Pilot Study of Schizophrenia. *Psychological Medicine*, **24**, 133–144.

Marenco, S. and Weinberger, D. R. (2000). The neurodevelopmental hypothesis of schizophrenia: following a trail of evidence from cradle to grave. *Development and Psychopathology*, **12**, 501–527.

Marneros, A. (1984). Frequency of occurrence of Schneider's first rank symptoms in Schizophrenia. *European Archives of Psychiatry and Neurological Sciences*, **234**, 78–82.

(1988). Schizophrenic first-rank symptoms in organic mental disorders. *British Journal of Psychiatry*, **152**, 625–628.

(1999). *Handbuch der unipolaren und bipolaren Erkrankungen.* Stuttgart, New York: Thieme.

(2003). The schizoaffective phenomenon – the state of the art. *Acta Psychiatrica Scandinavica* (Suppl.) **418**, 29–33.

Marneros, A. and Angst, J., eds. (2000). *Bipolar Disorders. 100 Years After Manic-depressive Insanity.* Dordrecht, Boston, London: Kluwer.

Marneros, A. and Goodwin, F., eds. (2004). *Mixed States, Rapid Cycling and Atypical Bipolar Disorders.* Cambridge: Cambridge University Press.

Marneros, A. and Rohde, A. (1997). 'Residual states' in affective, schizoaffective and schizophrenic disorders. In *Dysthymia and the Spectrum of Chronic Depressions*, ed. S. Akiskal and G. B. Cassano. New York, London: Guilford Press, pp. 75–86.

Marneros, A. and Tsuang, M. T., eds. (1986). *Schizoaffective Psychoses.* Berlin: Springer.

Marneros, A., Andreasen, N. C. and Tsuang, M. T. (1995a). *Psychotic Continuum.* Berlin, Heidelberg, New York: Springer.

Marneros, A., Deister, A. and Rohde, A. (1988a). Syndrome shift in the long-term course of schizoaffective disorders. *European Archives of Psychiatry and Neurological Sciences*, **238**, 97–104.

(1989a). Unipolar and bipolar schizoaffective disorders: a comparative study: I. Premorbid and sociodemographic features. *European Archives of Psychiatry and Neurological Sciences*, **239**, 158–163.

(1990a). The concept of distinct but voluminous groups of bipolar and unipolar diseases. I. Bipolar diseases. *European Archives of Psychiatry and Clinical Neuroscience*, **240**, 77–84.

(1990b). The concept of distinct but voluminous groups of bipolar and unipolar diseases. III. Bipolar and unipolar comparison. *European Archives of Psychiatry and Clinical Neuroscience*, **240**, 90–95.

(1991a). Autarkie und Autarkiebeeinträchtigung bei schizophrenen Patienten. *Nervenarzt*, **62**, 41–48.

(1991b). *(English abstract) Affektive, schizoaffektive und schizophrene Psychosen.* Berlin: Springer.

(1991c). Stability of diagnoses in affective, schizoaffective and schizophrenic disorders. Cross-sectional versus longitudinal diagnosis. *European Archives of Psychiatry and Clinical Neuroscience*, **241**, 187–192.

Marneros, A., Deister, A., Rohde, A., Jünemann, H. and Fimmers, R. (1988b). Long-term course of schizoaffective disorders. Part I: Definitions, methods, frequency of episodes and cycles. *European Archives of Psychiatry and Neurological Sciences*, **237**, 264–275.

Marneros, A., Pierschkalla, U., Rohde, A., Fischer, J. and Schmitz, K. (1994). Die Vorgeschichte alkoholkranker Straftäter, untergebracht nach § 64 StGB. *Monatsschrift für Kriminologie*, **77**, 13–22.

Marneros, A., Pillmann, F., Balzuweit, S., Blöink, R. and Haring, A. (2003). What is schizophrenic in ATPD? *Schizophrenia Bulletin*, **29**, 311–323.

Marneros, A., Pillmann, F., Haring, A. and Balzuweit, S. (2000). Die akuten vorübergehenden psychotischen Störungen. *Fortschritte der Neurologie-Psychiatrie*, **68**, S22–S25.

Marneros, A., Pillmann, F., Haring, A., Balzuweit, S. and Blöink, R. (2002a). The relation of 'acute and transient psychotic disorder' (ICD-10 F23) to bipolar schizoaffective disorder. *Journal of Psychiatric Research*, **36**, 165–171.

Marneros, A., Rohde, A. and Deister, A. (1989b). Unipolar and bipolar schizoaffective disorders: a comparative study. II. Long-term course. *European Archives of Psychiatry and Neurological Sciences*, **239**, 164–170.

(1995b). Psychotic continuum under longitudinal considerations. In *Psychotic Continuum*, ed. A. Marneros, N. C. Andreasen and M. T. Tsuang. Berlin, Heidelberg, New York: Springer, pp. 17–30.

(1998). Frequency and phenomenology of persisting alterations in affective, schizoaffective and schizophrenic disorders: a comparison. *Psychopathology*, **31**, 23–28.

Marneros, A., Rohde, A., Deister, A., Fimmers, R. and Jünemann, H. (1988c). Long-term course of schizoaffective disorders. Part III: Onset, type of episodes and syndrome shift, precipitating factors, suicidality, seasonality, inactivity of illness, and outcome. *European Archives of Psychiatry and Neurological Sciences*, **237**, 283–290.

Marneros, A., Rohde, A., Deister, A. and Sakamoto, K. (1987). Kurt Schneider's schizophrenia – the picture of schizophrenia in a Schneider-oriented university clinic. *Japanese Journal of Psychiatry and Neurology*, **41**, 171–178.

Marneros, A., Rohde, A., Deister, A. and Steinmeyer, E. M. (1989c). Prämorbide und soziale Merkmale von Patienten mit schizoaffektiven Psychosen. *Fortschritte der Neurologie-Psychiatrie*, **57**, 205–212.

(1990c). Behinderung und Residuum bei schizoaffektiven Psychosen – Daten, methodische Probleme und Hinweise für die zukünftige Forschung. *Fortschritte der Neurologie-Psychiatrie*, **58**, 66–75.

(1990). *Affective and Schizoaffective Disorders*. Berlin: Springer.

Marneros, A., Ullrich, S. and Rössner, D. (2002b). *Angeklagte Straftäter. Das Dilemma der Begutachtung*. Baden-Baden: Nomos.

Mattsson, B. and Perris, C. (1973). Cycloid psychoses: aspects of therapy and possible prevention of relapses. *Nordisk Psykiatrisk Tidsskrift*, **27**, 386–391.

Mayer-Gross, W. (1924). *Selbstschilderung und Verwirrtheit. Die oneiroide Erlebnisform*. Berlin: Springer.

McCabe, M. S. and Cadoret, R. J. (1976). Genetic investigations of atypical psychoses. I. Morbidity in parents and siblings. *Comprehensive Psychiatry*, **17**, 347–352.

McCabe, M. S. and Strömgren, E. (1975). Reactive psychoses: a family study. *Archives of General Psychiatry*, **32**, 447–454.

McCrae, R. R. and Costa, P. (1990). *Personality in Adulthood*. New York: Guilford Press.

McGorry, P. D., Yung, A. and Phillips, L. (2001). Ethics and early intervention in psychosis: keeping up the pace and staying in step. *Schizophrenia Research*, **51**, 17–29.

McGuffin, P., Farmer, A. and Harvey, I. (1991). A polydiagnostic application of operational criteria in studies of psychotic illness. Development and reliability of the OPCRIT system. *Archives of General Psychiatry*, **48**, 764–770.

McNeil, T. F., Cantor-Graae, E., Torrey, E. F. *et al.* (1994). Obstetric complications in histories of monozygotic twins discordant and concordant for schizophrenia. *Acta Psychiatrica Scandinavica*, **89**, 196–204.

Mechri, A., Gaha, L., Khammouma, S., Skhiri, T., Zaafrane, F. and Bedoui, A. (2000). Les psychoses aiguës nuptiales: à propos de 16 observations. *Encéphale*, **26**, 87–90.

Mellor, C. S. (1982). The present status of first-rank symptoms. *British Journal of Psychiatry*, **140**, 423–424.

Mellor, C. S., Sims, A. C. and Cope, R. V. (1981). Change of diagnosis in schizophrenia and first-rank symptoms: an eight-year follow-up. *Comprehensive Psychiatry*, **22**, 184–188.

Meltzer, H. Y. (1995). Psychotic continuum or disease entities: perspective from psychopharmacology. In *Psychotic Continuum*, ed. A. Marneros, N. C. Andreasen and M. T. Tsuang. Berlin, Heidelberg, New York: Springer, pp. 31–55.

Menezes, P. R., Rodrigues, L. C. and Mann, A. H. (1997). Predictors of clinical and social outcomes after hospitalization in schizophrenia. *European Archives of Psychiatry and Clinical Neuroscience*, **247**, 137–145.

Mitsuda, H. (1965). The concept of 'atypical psychosis' from the aspect of clinical genetics. *Acta Psychiatrica Scandinavica*, **41**, 372–377.

Mitsuda, H. and Fukuda, T. (1974). *Biological Mechanism of Schizophrenia and Schizophrenia-like Psychoses*. Tokyo: Igaku Shoin.

Mojtabai, R., Varma, V. K. and Susser, E. (2000). Duration of remitting psychoses with acute onset. Implications for ICD-10. *British Journal of Psychiatry*, **176**, 576–580.

Möller, H. J., Hohe-Schramm, M., Cording-Tommel, C. *et al.* (1989). The classification of functional psychoses and its implications for prognosis. *British Journal of Psychiatry*, **154**, 467–472.

Möller, H. J. and von Zerssen, D. (1986). *Der Verlauf schizophrener Psychosen unter den gegenwärtigen Behandlungsbedingungen*. Berlin, Heidelberg, New York: Springer.

Monroe, R. (1959). Episodic behavioral disorders – schizophrenia or epilepsy. *Archives of General Psychiatry*, **1**, 205–214.

Monroe, R. R. and Mickle, W. A. (1967). Alpha chloralose-activated electroencephalograms in psychiatric patients. *Journal of Nervous and Mental Disease*, **144**, 59–68.

Morel, B. A. (1857). *Traité des dégénérescences physiques, intellectuelles et morales de l'espèce humaine et des causes que produisent ces variétés maladives*. Paris: J. B. Baillière.

Mundt, C. (1982). Die schizophrene Primärpersönlichkeit im Lichte psychopathologischer und tiefenpsychologischer Ansätze. In *Psychopathologische Konzepte der Gegenwart*, ed. W. Janzarik. Stuttgart: Enke, pp. 158–166.

   (1985). *Das Apathiesyndrom der Schizophrenen*. Berlin, Heidelberg, New York, Tokyo: Springer.

   (1995). Psychotic continuum or distinct entities: perspectives from psychopathology. In *Psychotic Continuum*, ed. A. Marneros, N. C. Andreasen and M. T. Tsuang. Berlin, Heidelberg, New York: Springer, pp. 7–15.

Mundt, C., Backenstrass, M., Kronmüller, K. T., Fiedler, P., Kraus, A. and Stanghellini, G. (1997). Personality and endogenous/major depression: an empirical approach to typus melancholicus. 2. Validation of typus melancholicus core-properties by personality inventory scales. *Psychopathology*, **30**, 130–139.

Mundt, C., Reck, C., Backenstrass, M., Kronmüller, K. and Fiedler, P. (2000). Reconfirming the role of life events for the timing of depressive episodes. A two-year prospective follow-up study. *Journal of Affective Disorders*, **59**, 23–30.

Munk-Jørgensen, P. (1985). The schizophrenia diagnosis in Denmark. A register-based investigation. *Acta Psychiatrica Scandinavica*, **72**, 266–273.

   (1987). First-admission rates and marital status of schizophrenics. *Acta Psychiatrica Scandinavica*, **76**, 210–216.

Munk-Jørgensen, P. and Ewald, H. (2001). Epidemiology in neurobiological research: exemplified by the influenza–schizophrenia theory. *British Journal of Psychiatry* (Suppl.) **40**, s30–s32.

Murai, T., Toichi, M. and Sengoku, A. (1996). Functional psychosis mimicking acute confusional state: longitudinal neuropsychological assessment of an acute and transient psychotic patient. *Psychiatry and Clinical Neurosciences*, **50**, 257–260.

Murray, R. M. (1994). Neurodevelopmental schizophrenia: the rediscovery of dementia praecox. *British Journal of Psychiatry* (Suppl.) 6–12.

Nasrallah, H. A. (1993). Neurodevelopmental pathogenesis of schizophrenia. *Psychiatric Clinics of North America*, **16**, 269–280.

Neele, E. (1949). *Die phasischen Psychosen nach ihrem Erscheinungs- und Erbbild.* Leipzig: Barth.

Neumann, J. and Schulze, H. A. F. (1966). Psychopharmakologische Erfahrungen mit Methophenazin unter besonderer Berücksichtigung der Aufteilung der endogenen Psychosen nach Leonhard. *Psychiatrie, Neurologie und Medizinische Psychologie*, **1**, 11–17.

Ngoma, M. and Mbungu, M. (2000). Un bilan descriptif préliminaire de la bouffée délirante au Congo-Kinshasa. *Annales Médico-Psychologiques*, **158**, 483–491.

Niedermeyer, E. and Lopez da Silva, F. (1993). *Electroencephalography. Basic Principles, Clinical Applications, and Related Fields.* Baltimore, ML: Williams and Wilkins.

Novac, A. (1998). Atypical antipsychotics as enhancement therapy in rapid cycling mood states: a case study. *Annals of Clinical Psychiatry*, **10**, 107–111.

Offord, D. R., Abrams, N., Allen, N. and Poushinsky, M. (1979). Broken homes, parental psychiatric illness, and female delinquency. *American Journal of Orthopsychiatry*, **49**, 252–264.

Okasha, A., El Dawla, A. S., Khalil, A. H. and Saad, A. (1993). Presentation of acute psychosis in an egyptian sample: a transcultural comparison. *Comprehensive Psychiatry*, **34**, 4–9.

Olin, S. C., Mednick, S. A., Cannon, T. *et al.* (1998). School teacher ratings predictive of psychiatric outcome 25 years later. *British Journal of Psychiatry* (Suppl.) **172**, 7–13.

Opjordsmoen, S. (2001). Reactive psychosis and other brief psychotic episodes. *Current Psychiatry Reports*, **3**, 338–341.

Overall, J. E. and Gorham, D. R. (1962). The brief psychiatric rating scale. *Psychological Reports*, **10**, 799–812.

Patterson, D. A. and Lee, M. S. (1995). Field trial of the Global Assessment of Functioning Scale – Modified. *American Journal of Psychiatry*, **152**, 1386–1388.

Pauleikhoff, B. (1969). Atypische Psychosen. In *Schizophrenie und Zyklothymie*, ed. G. Huber. Stuttgart: Thieme.

Paykel, E. S. (1990). Life events in affective and schizoaffective disorders. In *Affective and Schizoaffective Disorders*, ed. A. Marneros and M. T. Tsuang. Berlin: Springer, pp. 107–122.

  (1994). Life events, social support and depression. *Acta Psychiatrica Scandinavica* (Suppl.), **377**, 50–58.

Perris, C. (1973). Cycloid psychoses: problems of etiology with special reference to genetic aspects. *Nordisk Psykiatrisk Tidsskrift*, **27**, 379–385.

  (1974). A study of cycloid psychosis. *Acta Psychiatrica Scandinavica* (Suppl.), **253**, 1–77.

  (1978). Morbidity suppressive effect of lithium carbonate in cycloid psychosis. *Archives of General Psychiatry*, **35**, 328–331.

(1986). The case for the independence of cycloid psychotic disorder from the schizoaffective disorders. In *Schizoaffective Psychoses*, ed. A. Marneros and M. T. Tsuang. Berlin, Heidelberg: Springer, pp. 272–308.

(1988). The concept of cycloid psychotic disorder. *Psychiatric Developments*, 1, 37–56.

Perris, C. and Brockington, I. F. (1981). Cycloid psychoses and their relation to the major psychoses. In *Biological Psychiatry*, ed. C. Perris, G. Struwe and B. Jansson. Amsterdam: Elsevier, pp. 447–450.

Perris, C. and Eisemann, M. (1989). Zykloide psychotische Störungen: Ihre Beziehung zu den schizoaffektiven Psychosen. In *Schizoaffektive Psychosen*, ed. A. Marneros. Berlin: Springer, pp. 29–43.

Perris, C. and Perris, H. (1978). Status within the family and early life experiences in patients with affective disorders and cycloid psychosis. *Psychiatria Clinica*, 11, 155–162.

Perris, C. and Smigan, L. (1984). The use of lithium in the longterm morbidity suppressive treatment of cycloid and schizoaffective psychoses. In *Psychiatry: The State of the Art, Vol. 3 Pharmacopsychiatry*, ed. P. Pichot. New York: Plenum, pp. 375–380.

Perris, C., Strandman, E. and Wahlby, L. (1979). HL-A antigens and the response to prophylactic lithium. *Neuropsychobiology*, 5, 114–118.

Pfuhlmann, B. (1998). Das Konzept der zykloiden Psychosen. *Fortschritte der Neurologie-Psychiatrie*, 66, 1–9.

Pfuhlmann, B., Franzek, E., Beckmann, H. and Stöber, G. (1999). Long-term course and outcome of severe postpartum psychiatric disorders. *Psychopathology*, 32, 192–202.

Pfuhlmann, B., Stöber, G., Franzek, E. and Beckmann, H. (1998). Cycloid psychoses predominate in severe postpartum psychiatric disorders. *Journal of Affective Disorders*, 50, 125–134.

Pichot, P. (1979). Les bouffées délirantes et les délires chroniques. Deux concepts nosologiques français. *Annales Medico-Psychologiques*, 137, 52–58.

(1982). The diagnosis and classification of mental disorders in French-speaking countries: background, current views and comparison with other nomenclatures. *Psychological Medicine*, 12, 475–492.

(1986a). A comparison of different national concepts of schizoaffective psychosis. In *Schizoaffective Psychoses*, ed. A. Marneros and M. T. Tsuang. Berlin, Heidelberg: Springer, pp. 8–17.

(1986b). The concept of 'bouffée délirante' with special reference to the Scandinavian concept of reactive psychosis. *Psychopathology*, 19, 35–43.

Pillmann, F. and Marneros, A. (2001). Carl Wernicke – Wirkung und Nachwirkung. *Fortschritte der Neurologie-Psychiatrie*, 69, 488–494.

(2003). Brief and acute psychoses: the development of concepts. *History of Psychiatry*, 14, 161–177.

Pillmann, F., Arndt, T., Ehrt, U., Haring, A., Kumbier, E. and Marneros, A. (2000a). An analysis of Wernicke's original case records: his contribution to the concept of cycloid psychoses. *History of Psychiatry*, 11, 355–369.

Pillmann, F., Schlote, K., Broich, K. and Marneros, A.(2000b). Electroencephalogram alterations during treatment with olanzapine. *Psychopharmacology (Berl.)*, 150, 216–219.

Pillmann, F., Haring, A., Balzuweit, S. and Marneros, A. (2001). Concordance of acute and transient psychotic disorders and cycloid psychoses. *Psychopathology*, 34, 305–311.

(2002). The concordance of ICD-10 acute and transient psychosis and DSM-IV brief psychotic disorder. *Psychological Medicine*, **32**, 525–533.

Pillmann, F., Haring, A., Balzuweit, S., Blöink, R. and Marneros, A. (2003). Bouffée délirante and ICD-10 acute and transient psychoses: a comparative study. *Australian and New Zealand Journal of Psychiatry*, **37**, 327–333.

Pitta, J. C. and Blay, S. L. (1997). Psychogenic (reactive) and hysterical psychoses: a cross-system reliability study. *Acta Psychiatrica Scandinavica*, **95**, 112–118.

Procci, W. R. (1976). Schizo-affective psychosis: fact or fiction? A survey of the literature. *Archives of General Psychiatry*, **33**, 1167–1178.

Pull, C. B., Pull, M. C. and Pichot, P. (1983). Nosological position of schizo-affective psychoses in France. *Psychiatria Clinica*, **16**, 141–148.

(1984). Des critères empiriques français pour les psychoses. I. Position du problème et méthodologie. *Encéphale*, **10**, 119–123.

(1987). Des critères empiriques français pour les psychoses. II. Consensus des psychiatres français et définitions provisoires. *Encéphale*, **13**, 53–57.

Rachlin, H. L. (1935). A follow-up study of Hoch's benign stupor cases. *American Journal of Psychiatry*, **92**, 531–558.

Radomsky, E. D., Haas, G. L., Mann, J. J. and Sweeney, J. A. (1999). Suicidal behavior in patients with schizophrenia and other psychotic disorders. *American Journal of Psychiatry*, **156**, 1590–1595.

Remington, G., Menuck, M., Schmidt, P. and Legault, S. (1990). The remitting atypical psychoses: clinical and nosologic considerations. *Canadian Journal of Psychiatry*, **35**, 36–40.

Riecher-Rössler, A. and Rössler, W. (1998). The course of schizophrenic psychoses: what do we really know? A selective review from an epidemiological perspective. *European Archives of Psychiatry and Clinical Neuroscience*, **248**, 189–202.

Riecher-Rössler, A., Fatkenheuer, B., Löffler, W., Maurer, K. and Häfner, H. (1992). Is age of onset in schizophrenia influenced by marital status? Some remarks on the difficulties and pitfalls in the systematic testing of a 'simple' question. *Social Psychiatry and Psychiatric Epidemiology*, **27**, 122–128.

Ring, N., Tantam, D., Montague, L., Newby, D., Black, D. and Morris, J. (1991). Gender differences in the incidence of definite schizophrenia and atypical psychosis – focus on negative symptoms of schizophrenia. *Acta Psychiatrica Scandinavica*, **84**, 489–496.

Ritsher, J. E., Warner, V., Johnson, J. G. and Dohrenwend, B. P. (2001). Inter-generational longitudinal study of social class and depression: a test of social causation and social selection models. *British Journal of Psychiatry* (Suppl.), **40**, s84–s90.

Robins, E. and Guze, S. B. (1970). Establishment of diagnostic validity in psychiatric illness: its application to schizophrenia. *American Journal of Psychiatry*, **126**, 983–987.

Robinson, D. G., Woerner, M. G., Alvir, J. M. *et al.* (1999). Predictors of treatment response from a first episode of schizophrenia or schizoaffective disorder. *American Journal of Psychiatry*, **156**, 544–549.

Rohde, A. and Marneros, A. (1992). Schizoaffective disorders with and without onset in the puerperium. *European Archives of Psychiatry and Clinical Neuroscience*, **242**, 27–33.

Roth, M. and McClelland, H. (1979). The relationship of 'nuclear' and 'atypical' psychoses. *Psychiatria Clinica*, **12**, 23–54.

Röttig, S. (2001). EEG-Befunde bei nach ICD-10 diagnostizierten akuten vorübergehenden, schizoaffektiven und schizophrenen Psychosen (Thesis). Halle: Martin-Luther-Universität Halle-Wittenberg.

Rouchouse, J. C. (1996). Analyse ethopsychophysiologique d'une bouffée délirante. Récit auto-biographique et position de la bouffée délirante parmi les psychoses. *Annales Médico-Psychologiques*, **154**, 10–19.

Sajith, S. G., Chandrasekaran, R., Sadanandan Unni, K. E. and Sahai, A. (2002). Acute polymorphic psychotic disorder: diagnostic stability over 3 years. *Acta Psychiatrica Scandinavica*, **105**, 104–109.

Sakado, K., Sato, T., Uehara, T., Sato, S., Sakado, M. and Kumagai, K. (1997). Evaluating the diagnostic specificity of the Munich Personality Test dimensions in major depression. *Journal of Affective Disorders*, **43**, 187–194.

Saletu, B. (1992). Pharmako-EEG. In *Neuro-Psychopharmaka. Ein Therapiehandbuch, Band 1: Allgemeine Grundlagen der Psychopharmakotherapie*, ed. P. Riederer, G. Laux and W. Pöldinger. Wien, New York: Springer, pp. 89–108.

Saletu, B., Anderer, P., Kinsperger, K. and Grünberger, J. (1987). Topographic brain mapping of EEG in neuropsychopharmacology – Part II. Clinical applications (pharmaco EEG imaging). *Methods and Findings in Experimental and Clinical Pharmacology*, **9**, 385–408.

Sartorius, N., Gulbinat, W., Harrison, G., Laska, E. and Siegel, C. (1996). Long-term follow-up of schizophrenia in 16 countries. A description of the International Study of Schizophrenia conducted by the World Health Organization. *Social Psychiatry and Psychiatric Epidemiology*, **31**, 249–258.

Sartorius, N., Üstün, T. B., Korten, A., Cooper, J. E. and van Drimmelen, J. (1995). Progress toward achieving a common language in psychiatry, II: results from the international field trials of the ICD-10 diagnostic criteria for research for mental and behavioral disorders. *American Journal of Psychiatry*, **152**, 1427–1437.

Sauer, H., Richter, P., Czernik, A. *et al.* (1997). Personality differences between patients with major depression and bipolar disorder – the impact of minor symptoms on self-ratings of personality. *Journal of Affective Disorders*, **42**, 169–177.

Saury, H. (1886). *Etude clinique sur la folie héréditaire (les dégénérés)*. Paris: Delahaye/Lescrosnier.

Schär, V., Zeit, T., Heinemann, F. and Otto, H. (1995). Zur Hypofrontalität im 99m-Tc-HMPOA-SPECT bei 'akuten' Psychosen. *Nervenheilkunde*, **14**, 379–384.

Schneider, K. (1950). *Klinische Psychopathologie*. Stuttgart: Thieme.

(1959). *Clinical Psychopathology*. New York: Grune & Stratton.

Schöpf, J. and Rust, B. (1994a). Follow-up and family study of postpartum psychoses. Part I: overview. *European Archives of Psychiatry and Clinical Neuroscience*, **244**, 101–111.

Schöpf, J. and Rust, B. (1994b). Follow-up and family study of postpartum psychoses. Part IV: schizophreniform psychoses and brief reactive psychoses: lack of nosological relation to schizophrenia. *European Archives of Psychiatry and Clinical Neuroscience*, **244**, 141–144.

Schröder, P. (1918). Ungewöhnliche periodische Psychosen. *Monatsschrift für Psychiatrie und Neurologie*, **44**, 44.

(1920). Degeneratives Irresein und Degenerationspsychosen. *Zeitschrift für die gesamte Neurologie und Psychiatrie*, **60**, 119–126.

(1922). Degenerationspsychosen und Dementia praecox. *Archiv für Psychiatrie und Nervenkrankheiten,* **66,** 1–51.

(1926). Über Degenerationspsychosen (Metabolische Erkrankungen). *Zeitschrift für die gesamte Neurologie und Psychiatrie,* **105,** 539–547.

Schubart, C. (1986). *Schizophrenie und soziale Anpassung: eine prospektive Längsschnittuntersuchung.* Berlin: Springer.

Schubart, C., Krumm, B., Biehl, H. and Schwarz, R. (1986). Measurement of social disability in a schizophrenic patient group. Definition, assessment and outcome over 2 years in a cohort of schizophrenic patients of recent onset. *Social Psychiatry,* **21,** 1–9.

Schwartz, J. E., Fennig, S., Tanenberg-Karant, M. *et al.* (2000). Congruence of diagnoses 2 years after a first-admission diagnosis of psychosis. *Archives of General Psychiatry,* **57,** 593–600.

Shenton, M. E., Dickey, C. C., Frumin, M. and McCarley, R. W. (2001). A review of MRI findings in schizophrenia. *Schizophrenia Research,* **49,** 1–52.

Shorter, E. (1997). *A History of Psychiatry: From the Era of the Asylum to the Age of Prozac.* New York: John Wiley.

Sieber, M. F. and Angst, J. (1990). Alcohol, tobacco and cannabis: 12-year longitudinal associations with antecedent social context and personality. *Drug and Alcohol Dependence,* **25,** 281–292.

Sigmund, D. and Mundt, C. (1999). The cycloid type and its differentiation from core schizophrenia: a phenomenological approach. *Comprehensive Psychiatry,* **40,** 4–18.

Simpson, T. L. and Miller, W. R. (2002). Concomitance between childhood sexual and physical abuse and substance use problems. A review. *Clinical Psychology Review,* **22,** 27–77.

Singer, L., Ebtinger, R. and Mantz, H. (1980). Le devenir des bouffées délirantes. Étude catamnestique de 74 cas. *Annales Médico-Psychologiques,* **138,** 1097–1106.

Singer, L., Roos, L., Danion, J. M. and Heidet, S. (1986). Bouffées délirantes et schizophrénie. Étude catamnestique comparative de deux groupes de patients. *Annales Médico-Psychologiques,* **144,** 1029–1043.

Smith, G. N., Flynn, S. W., Kopala, L. C. *et al.* (1997). A comprehensive method of assessing routine CT scans in schizophrenia. *Acta Psychiatrica Scandinavica,* **96,** 395–401.

Snyder, S., Goodpaster, W. A., Pitts, W. M., Jr., Pokorny, A. D. and Gustin, Q. L. (1985). Demography of psychiatric patients with borderline personality traits. *Psychopathology,* **18,** 38–49.

Staehelin, J. E. (1931). Über die Entstehung periodischer Geistesstörungen. *Schweizer Archiv für Neurologie, Neurochirurgie und Psychiatrie,* **27,** 354–361.

(1946). Zur Frage der Emotionspsychosen. *Bulletin der Schweizer Akademie der Medizinischen Wissenschaften,* **2,** 121–130.

Stanghellini, G. and Mundt, C. (1997). Personality and endogenous/major depression: an empirical approach to typus melancholicus. 1. Theoretical issues. *Psychopathology,* **30,** 119–129.

Stastny, P., Perlick, D., Zeavin, L., Empfield, M. and Mayer, M. (1984). Early parental absence as an indicator of course and outcome in chronic schizophrenia. *American Journal of Psychiatry,* **141,** 294–296.

Stephens, J. H., Richard, P. and McHugh, P. R. (1997). Long-term follow-up of patients hospitalized for schizophrenia, 1913 to 1940. *Journal of Nervous and Mental Disease,* **185,** 715–721.

Stevens, J. (1987). Brief psychoses: do they contribute to the good prognosis and equal prevalence of schizophrenia in developing countries? *British Journal of Psychiatry,* **151,** 393–396.

Stöber, G., Kocher, I., Franzek, E. and Beckmann, H. (1997). First-trimester maternal gestational infection and cycloid psychosis. *Acta Psychiatrica Scandinavica*, **96**, 319–324.

Störring, G. (1969). Zyklothymie, Emotionspsychosen, Schizophrenie. In *Schizophrenie und Zyklothymie*, ed. G. Huber. Stuttgart: Thieme, pp. 68–77.

Störring, G. E., Suchenwirth, R. and Völkel, H. (1962). Emotionalität und cycloide Psychosen. *Psychiatrie, Neurologie und Medizinische Psychologie*, **14**, 85–97.

Strakowski, S. M. (1994). Diagnostic validity of schizophreniform disorder. *American Journal of Psychiatry*, **151**, 815–824.

Strauss, J. S. and Carpenter, W. T., Jr. (1972). The prediction of outcome in schizophrenia. I. Characteristics of outcome. *Archives of General Psychiatry*, **27**, 739–746.

(1974). The prediction of outcome in schizophrenia. II. Relationships between predictor and outcome variables: a report from the WHO international pilot study of schizophrenia. *Archives of General Psychiatry*, **31**, 37–42.

Strik, W. K., Dierks, T., Franzek, E., Maurer, K. and Beckmann, H. (1993). Differences in P300 amplitudes and topography between cycloid psychosis and schizophrenia in Leonhard's classification. *Acta Psychiatrica Scandinavica*, **87**, 179–183.

Strik, W. K., Fallgatter, A. J., Stoeber, G., Franzek, E. and Beckmann, H. (1997). Specific P300 features in patients with cycloid psychosis. *Acta Psychiatrica Scandinavica*, **95**, 67–72.

Strömgren, E. (1986). Reactive (psychogenic) psychoses and their relations to schizoaffective psychoses. In *Schizoaffective Psychoses*, ed. A. Marneros and M. T. Tsuang. Berlin, Heidelberg: Springer, pp. 260–271.

(1987). The development of the concept of reactive psychoses. *Psychopathology*, **20**, 62–67.

Strömgren, L. S. (1997). ECT in acute delirium and related clinical states. *Convulsive Therapy*, **13**, 10–17.

Susser, E. and Wanderling, J. (1994). Epidemiology of nonaffective acute remitting psychosis vs. schizophrenia: sex and sociocultural setting. *Archives of General Psychiatry*, **51**, 294–301.

Susser, E., Fennig, S., Jandorf, L., Amador, X. and Bromet, E. (1995a). Epidemiology, diagnosis and course of brief psychoses. *American Journal of Psychiatry*, **152**, 1743–1748.

Susser, E., Finnerty, M. T. and Sohler, N. (1996). Acute psychoses: a proposed diagnosis for ICD-11 and DSM-V. *Psychiatric Quarterly*, **67**, 165–176.

Susser, E., Varma, V. K., Malhotra, S., Conover, S. and Amador, X. F. (1995b). Delineation of acute and transient psychotic disorders in a developing country setting. *British Journal of Psychiatry*, **167**, 216–219.

Susser, E., Varma, V. K., Mattoo, S. K. *et al.* (1998). Long-term course of acute brief psychosis in a developing country setting. *British Journal of Psychiatry*, **173**, 226–230.

Tellenbach, H. (1976). *Melancholie, 3.Aufl.* Berlin: Springer.

Thara, R. and Srinivasan, T. N. (1997). Outcome of marriage in schizophrenia. *Social Psychiatry and Psychiatric Epidemiology*, **32**, 416–420.

Tien, A. Y. and Eaton, W. W. (1992). Psychopathologic precursors and sociodemographic risk factors for the schizophrenia syndrome. *Archives of General Psychiatry*, **49**, 37–46.

Torrey, E. F. and Bowler, A. E. (1990). The seasonality of schizophrenics births: A reply to Marc S. Lewis. *Schizophrenia Bulletin*, **16**, 1–3.

Torrey, E. F. and Torrey, B. B. (1980). Sex differences in the seasonality of schizophrenic births. *British Journal of Psychiatry*, **137**, 101.

Tsoh, J. M., Leung, H. C., Ungvari, G. S. and Lee, D. T. (2000). Brief acute psychosis following hysterectomy in ethnopsychiatric context. *Singapore Medical Journal*, **41**, 359–362.

Tsuang, M. T. (1978). Suicide in schizophrenics, manics, depressives, and surgical controls. A comparison with general population suicide mortality. *Archives of General Psychiatry*, **35**, 153–155.

   (1995). Psychotic continuum: perspectives from family studies. In *Psychotic Continuum*, ed. A. Marneros, N. C. Andreasen and M. T. Tsuang. Berlin, Heidelberg, New York: Springer, pp. 57–66.

Tsuang, M. T., Fleming, J. A. and Simpson, J. C. (1999). Suicide and Schizophrenia. In *The Harvard Medical School Guide to Suicide Assessment and Intervention*, ed. D. G. Jacobs. San Francisco: Jossey-Bass, pp. 287–299.

Tsuang, M. T., Tohen, M. and Zahner, G. E. P. (1995). *Textbook in Psychiatric Epidemiology*. New York: Wiley-Liss.

Tsuang, M. T., Winokur, G. and Crowe, R. R. (1980). Morbidity risks of schizophrenia and affective disorders among first degree relatives of patients with schizophrenia, mania, depression and surgical conditions. *British Journal of Psychiatry*, **137**, 497–504.

Tucker, G. J., Price, T. R., Johnson, V. B. and McAllister, T. (1986). Phenomenology of temporal lobe dysfunction: a link to atypical psychosis – a series of cases. *Journal of Nervous and Mental Disease*, **174**, 348–356.

Ungvari, G. (1985). Klinisch-genetische Untersuchungen im Rahmen der Leonhardschen Systematik. *Psychiatrie, Neurologie und Medizinische Psychologie*, **37**, 309–317.

Ungvari, G. S. and Mullen, P. E. (2000). Reactive psychoses revisited. *Australian and New Zealand Journal of Psychiatry*, **34**, 458–467.

Ungvari, G. S., Leung, H. C. and Tang, W. K. (2000). Reactive psychosis: a classical category nearing extinction? *Psychiatry and Clinical Neurosciences*, **54**, 621–624.

Vaillant, G. E. (1964). An historical review of the remitting schizophrenias. *Journal of Nervous and Mental Disease*, **138**, 48–56.

van Gülick-Bailer, M., Maurer, K. and Häfner, H., eds. (1995). *Schedules for Clinical Assessment in Neuropsychiatry*. Bern: Huber.

van Heeringen, K., Audenaert, K., Van de Wiele, L. and Verstraete, A. (2000). Cortisol in violent suicidal behaviour: association with personality and monoaminergic activity. *Journal of Affective Disorders*, **60**, 181–189.

van Kammen, D. P. (1995). Biochemical heterogeneiety in schizophrenia: implications and research strategies of the state dependency model. In *Psychotic Continuum*, ed. A. Marneros, N. C. Andreasen and M. T. Tsuang, Berlin, Heidelberg, New York: Springer, pp. 107–126.

Verma, V. K., Malhotra, S. and Jiloha, R. C. (1992). Acute non-organic psychotic state in India: symptomatology. *Indian Journal of Psychiatry*, **34**, 89–101.

Viinamaki, H., Niskanen, L., Jaaskelainen, J. *et al.* (1996). Factors predicting psychosocial recovery in psychiatric patients. *Acta Psychiatrica Scandinavica*, **94**, 365–371.

von Trostorff, S. (1968). Über die hereditäre Belastung bei den zykloiden Psychosen, den unsystematischen und systematischen Schizophrenien. *Psychiatrie, Neurologie und Medizinische Psychologie*, **20**, 98–106.

von Zerssen, D. (1976). Der 'Typus melancholicus' in psychometrischer Sicht. *Zeitschrift für klinische Psychologie und Psychotherapie*, **24**, 200–220.

(2001). Personality and Affective Disorders. In *Contemporary Psychiatry*, ed. F. Henn, N. Sartoruis, H. Helmchen and H. Lauter. Heidelberg: Springer. Volume 3, Part 1, pp. 279–298.

Watt, D. C. and Szulecka, T. K. (1979). The effect of sex, marriage and age at first admission on the hospitalization of schizophrenics during 2 years following discharge. *Psychological Medicine*, **9**, 529–539.

Wernicke, C. (1900). *Grundriss der Psychiatrie in klinischen Vorlesungen*. Leipzig: Thieme.

Wexler, B. E., Lyons, L., Lyons, H. and Mazure, C. M. (1997). Physical and sexual abuse during childhood and development of psychiatric illnesses during adulthood. *Journal of Nervous and Mental Disease*, **185**, 522–524.

Weygandt, W. (1899). *Über die Mischzustände des manisch-depressiven Irreseins*. München: Lehmann.

Wiersma, D., Giel, R., De Jong, A. and Slooff, C. J. (1983). Social class and schizophrenia in a Dutch cohort. *Psychological Medicine*, **13**, 141–150.

Wiersma, D., Nienhuis, F. J., Slooff, C. J. and Giel, R. (1998). Natural course of schizophrenic disorders: a 15-year follow-up of a Dutch incidence cohort. *Schizophrenia Bulletin*, **24**, 75–85.

Wiersma, D., Wanderling, J., Dragomirecka, E. *et al.* (2000). Social disability in schizophrenia: its development and prediction over 15 years in incidence cohorts in six European centres. *Psychological Medicine*, **30**, 1155–1167.

Wig, N. N. and Parhee, R. (1988). Acute and transient psychoses. A view from the developing countries. In *International Classification in Psychiatry*, ed. J. E. Mezzich and M. Cranach. Cambridge: Cambridge University Press, pp. 115–121.

Wing, J. K., Cooper, J. E. and Sartorius, N. (1974). *Measurement and Classification of Psychiatric Symptoms*. London: Cambridge University Press.

Winokur, G., Scharfetter, C. and Angst, J. (1985). Stability of psychotic symptomatology (delusions, hallucinations), affective syndromes, and schizophrenic symptoms (thought disorder, incongruent affect) over episodes in remitting psychoses. *European Archives of Psychiatry and Neurological Sciences*, **234**, 303–307.

World Health Organization (1979). *Schizophrenia: An International Follow-up Study*. Chichester: John Wiley.

(1992). *The ICD-10 Classification of Mental and Behavioral Disorders: Clinical Descriptions and Diagnostic Guidelines*. Geneva: WHO.

(1993). *The ICD-10 Classification of Mental and Behavioral Disorders: Diagnostic Criteria for Research*. Geneva: WHO.

Yamauchi, K., Ono, Y., Baba, K. and Ikegami, N. (2001). The actual process of rating the global assessment of functioning scale. *Comprehensive Psychiatry*, **42**, 403–409.

Zarate, C. A., Tohen, M. and Land, M. L. (2000). First-episode schizophreniform disorder: comparisons with first-episode schizophrenia. *Schizophrenia Research*, **46**, 31–34.

Zhang-Wong, J., Beiser, M., Bean, G. and Iacono, W. G. (1995). Five-year course of schizophreniform disorder. *Psychiatry Research*, **59**, 109–117.

Index